TO:

All the Best

Paddy Boyle

World

Champion

2009

Pure Grit

Paddy Doyle

Multi Guinness World Record Holder

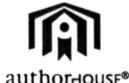
authorHOUSE®

AuthorHouse™ UK Ltd.
500 Avebury Boulevard
Central Milton Keynes, MK9 2BE
www.authorhouse.co.uk
Phone: 08001974150

© 2009 Paddy Doyle. All rights reserved.

No part of this book may be reproduced, stored in a retrieval system, or transmitted by any means without the written permission of the author.

First published by AuthorHouse 6/23/2009

ISBN: 978-1-4389-9541-0 (sc)

This book is printed on acid-free paper.

Contents

Foreword	1
The Powerful Mind	3
Introduction	5
The Beginning	7
German Challenge	11
Most Demanding World Records	15
World's Fittest Athlete Physical Fitness Challenge Record	34
Hard Times And Making Ends Meet	42
Wuma Warlords Kumite Challenge Record Title	55
Special Forces Speed March	60
Guinness World Records Festival, Flensburg, Germany	64
World Fitness Champions Record Title 27^h February 2006	68
Gleason's Boxing Gym Brooklyn New York 5 August 2006	71
Strength Step-Ups Carrying 56lb Back Pack	78
Martial ArtS And Boxing Punching World Records 19 January 2007	82
The Arden Cross Country Challenge Marathon 24 February 2007	85
World Record Breakers Cup Challenge 18 April - 2 May 2007	90

Guinness World Records Day 8 November 2007	95
Military Special Forces Training	108
Training And What Makes Me Tick	113
Stamina's Gym	117
Guinness World Records Day	122
Challengers And Jealous Talkers	125
Pushing It To The Limits	128
Letting Off Steam	133
Courses And Hobbies	138
Contacts And Friends	143
Doyle's World Record Total FitnEss Training Preparation Tips	147
Believing In Yourself	183
Great Times And What's Next	187
About The Author	189

DEDICATIONS

This book is dedicated to my loyal friends and training team; my fiancée Deborah Jayne Green, Jean Green, Trixie my dog, Paul Jones, David Chubb, Graham, Betty & Matthew Petrie, Colin Dickinson, Wayne Bernstein, Micky Roath, Deborah Ganderton, Bryan Vernum, Nigel Perry, Bryan Perry, Vince Brereton, Mark Dawes, osteopath John Williams and Joe Egan.

To the World Record Authorities and official Associations; Craig Glenday, Guinness World Records Editor; Laura Farmer, Guinness Records Manager; Alan Ashes, World Association of Special Forces; Richard Hopkins, WUMA President; Ralf Laue, Book of Alternative Records Editor, Dean Gould, President of Record Holders Registry UK; Dr David Adamovich, USA President of Registry of Record Holders & Editor of Believe the Unbelievable Book of Records; Chad Netherland, World Record Holder USA; Dale Harder, Book of Strength Speed Records Editor; Paul Skousen, Book of World Record Editor; Andrew Simms, Soldier Magazine Editor; Simon Steele, Leamington Courier Sports Editor; Aidan Carroll Senior Self Defence Coach, Corner Stone Karate Club, and to Valerie Ball who edited the original manuscript.

To my sponsors Tony and Maggie Ryan, MarCity Developments; Jim Mosley, Co-op Construction Birmingham; Joe Lynch, Liverpool Night Club Owner; UK Gear British Army fitness training suppliers; Mack Birmingham Market wholesale suppliers; Thienna Ho Products USA; Wayne Hubball; To Professor and Author, Dr Carl Chinn,

Malcolm Boyden BBC Radio Presenter ; Bob Brolly BBC Radio Presenter ; Birmingham Evening Mail newspaper for their continued support; BBC Radio West Midlands; Titan films UK, Solihull Observer newspaper… and last but not least, the army units I served with, who taught me direction, discipline and respect.

www.worldsfittestathlete.co.uk

FOREWORD

Paddy Doyle? The Guinness World Fitness Endurance Champion? He's certainly no looker! As far as I can recall, I first met Paddy in a dark, backstreet martial arts boxing gym in the East End of London. This dive of a place, under the arches of a train line, seemed a fitting place to meet a bloke who happened to be a right bruiser, a broken-nosed, cauliflower-eared meat-head of a club bouncer. By the end of our session (a photographic assignment, I hasten to add, not a fight!) I realized my initial prejudices were ridiculous and unfounded... I was in the presence of a true athlete and, above all, a real gentleman.

So I give you Paddy Doyle, the World's Fittest Athlete and probably with genuine justification. When we established the Guinness World Records Fitness Challenge, to ascertain who could be the fastest to perform a series of excruciating fitness trials – such as a 12-mile run, 12-mile speed march carrying a 40lbs back pack, 1,250 push- ups, 3,250 sit-up crunches, 1,250 hip flexors (lifting 10lbs weight), 110-mile cycle, 20-mile row, 20-mile cross trainer, weights lifted 300,000lbs, 2-mile swim, and 1,250 star jumps… who would step up to the plate and set the benchmark for the record? Paddy Doyle. (He finished in an incredible 18 hrs, 56 mins, 9 secs.)

Paddy Doyle, the holder of many Guinness World

Record Titles. For me, it's almost impossible to sum up this humorous, gentle, generous and unrivalled powerhouse of a man in just a simple word. There's so much more to him than showing off his determination with a simple push-up.

If I had to choose one word, I'd look back in Guinness World Records history, to the great Roy Castle, presenter of the fantastically inspirational Record Breakers TV Show, and say 'dedication' which could have been coined to describe our Paddy. His dedication to be the best in the world, to help and support others in the earlier part of his career, to raise money for charity and to push himself beyond his own expectations is what defines him. Can there be more a dedicated record holder than Paddy? He's certainly in the highest echelons of our highest achievers.

Paddy once told me that if it were not for Guinness World Records, he'd more than likely have faced a lifetime at Her Majesty's pleasure. And while you can thank us for keeping Paddy out of trouble, he is responsible for enriching our book each year, and inspiring children – and adults – across the world to set themselves goals, dedicate themselves to achieving them, and then setting more impossible goals in the future.

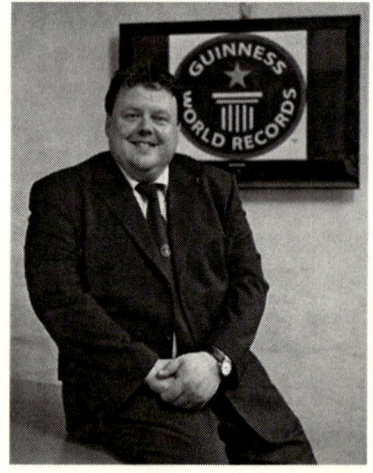

Craig Glenday
Guinness World
Records Editor 2009.

THE POWERFUL MIND

Within the context of Birmingham as a community that is home to almost a million people, you might think of Paddy Doyle's achievements as interesting if insignificant. You'd be wrong. Admired for the limits to which he stretches his body in pursuit of endurance records, the former paratrooper's success is based on a principle from which all of us, whether young or old, active or infirm, could draw inspiration and benefit. Above all, Doyle believes the body won't reach its potential until the mind has accepted what is possible first. Thus, to him, the pain barrier which most of us associate with physical effort is but a stage on the way to the ultimate achievement.

He translates that to his students and strength athlete followers by insisting that 'if you can be successful in the gym, you can be successful in life.' The point is no less relevant to the rest of us. Look at the newspapers on any day of the week and you will read about a person, issue or concern where attitude is a key ingredient. The closest that most people come to meeting Paddy's principles is an occasional display of will-power. Absorb the 'mind over matter' and you can start to realise the waste of potential in our own lives. The whole point is the power of the mind, and what

Paddy has shown throughout his athletic career is that if you can focus and control the mind, you can achieve your goals.

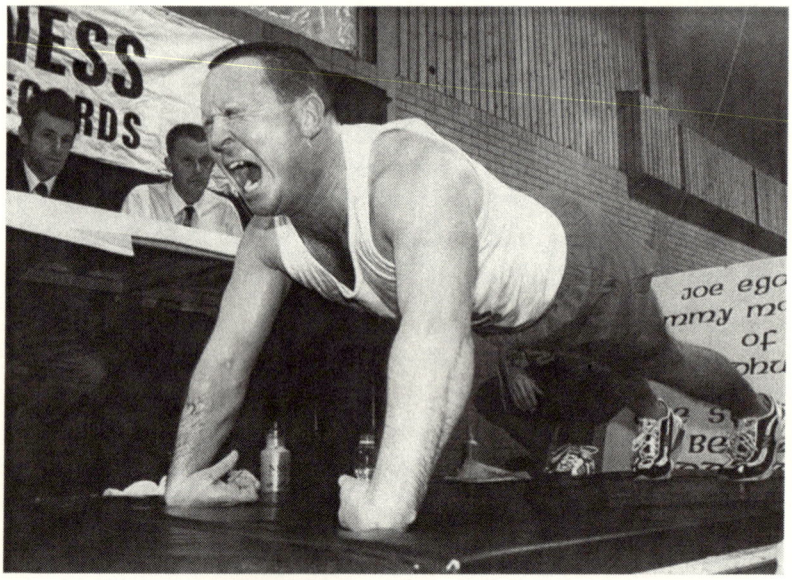

{The first Guinness World Record attempt for the most strict back of hands push ups in 1 hour, total 660. Date 5th March 2000. B'ham UK}

INTRODUCTION

Ranked 'Guinness Fitness Endurance Champion,' he has broken a staggering career total of 172 Course, Regional, National, British, European and World strength speed stamina records around the globe. In the eyes of his many thousands of admirers he is a true legend... a sporting phenomenon. The Midlands based 'World Endurance Athlete' has devoted his life to an inextinguishable passion for sport. But what makes him tick? What turns him on and keeps him going?

In *Pure Grit*, the gritty ex-paratrooper and Black Belt 3 DAN martial arts instructor talks of his traumatic and troublesome past which he had to go through to become the World's Number One for holding the most fitness records under several different sporting categories. He describes how he transformed his world from that of a 16 year old teenage tearaway to a sporting great.

He outlines his heroic athletic conquests, his hopes for the future, his dearest wishes ... and his worst fears.

Pure Grit investigates the magnificent mental attitude of the world's undisputed stamina endurance king, and visits Paddy Doyle's shrine... a spit and sawdust gymnasium in a Birmingham suburb, where the toughest of the tough are reduced to sweat, blood and tears. Qualified professionals from the sporting world will give their opinions and scientific evidence of why he has a remarkable thirst for pushing his body to the ultimate limits of endurance. Some of the world's most famous athletes look up to Paddy Doyle as an amazing example. They all admire him. but they know they can never beat him. For the first time his mental approach, life experiences and training secrets will be uncovered in ***Pure Grit***.

THE BEGINNING

As a young boy I was always prepared to have a go at all sports, representing my Judo club in the Midlands Junior Judo Championships and winning bronze and silver medals. I then started gymnastics and athletics, representing my senior school at regional level. However, my first secondary school was not for me, I was not learning anything at all, the standard of education was very poor. My father took me out of the school and managed to get me into St Edmund Campion secondary school, I was known amongst my friends as a rebellious teenager, sometimes fighting in the playground and outside the school gates when school had finished. I never backed out of a scuffle. As I was coming to the end of my schooldays, the hunger for more violence escalated and I found myself getting caught up in street fights with grown men. Between the ages of sixteen and eighteen, all I seemed to do was drink, fight and create havoc everywhere I went. I then turned to amateur boxing which I stuck at for four years, fighting at welterweight. Other boxers and I would fight at interclub tournaments in the Midlands. I have to admit I was late developing my boxing skills and techniques. My method was to come out all guns blazing, which did not work for my first two fights. I clearly remember getting my nose broken when I had my first fight, and losing on points to a London boxer. I should have won that fight easily, but brawn and not brains took over.

Between the ages of eighteen and twenty I had many confrontations with organized gangs until I decided enough was enough and at the age of twenty-one I joined the regular army, serving in the 2nd Battalion Parachute Regiment.

I was awarded the Champion Recruit Trophy for outstanding hard work, but the devil was still inside me. When the weekends came I was caught up in street fights with other soldiers from different regiments in Aldershot, and, being a regular visitor to the glasshouse (army jail) I was discharged from the army in 1986. My Commanding Officer said in his report, 'Private Doyle has an unacceptably aggressive nature. He lacks the ability to back away from a situation in which he finds himself in conflict. In such circumstances he becomes uncontrollable and tries to find a release by offering physical violence, irrespective of the rank of those involved.'

In 1987 I started my first part-time club teaching street self defence, boxing and fitness endurance training. As I was improving my own levels of stamina, I wanted to push my body further to extreme limits. I have mentioned many times that my competitive sporting career started with an old edition of the Guinness Book of Records. I never realised that it was to take me on a journey to achieving a career total of 172 Course, Regional, National, British, European and World fitness, endurance, Martial Arts, and Boxing title records.

But I am still competing in a minority sport where sponsorship is hard to find, and money is hard to come by. I have been approached to sort out individuals' problems... for instance, if they were being hassled, bullied, or threatened. But that is the sort of person I am; willing to help certain people out if they are genuinely in the right, giving me a financial handshake in return. I hope I am now a good role model. It is up to you to decide when you have read my book.

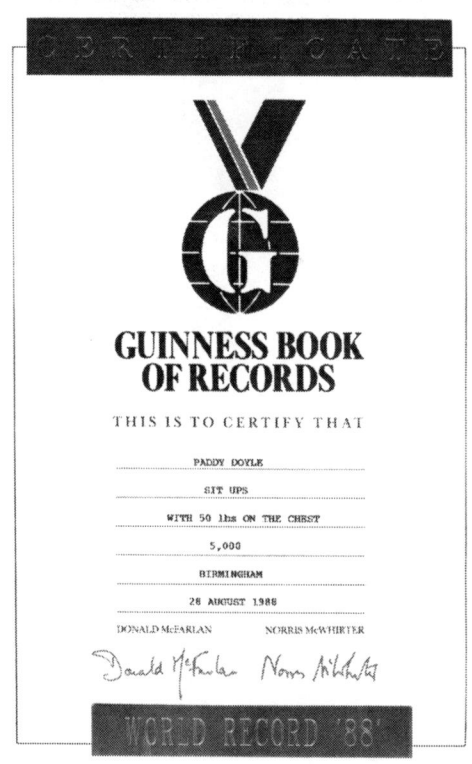

NW HERALD, Friday, March 5, 1999

Paddy on top of the world again

ATHERSTONE endurance world record holder Paddy Doyle has won another world martial arts title after a gruelling eight fights in two weeks.

Paddy claimed the World United Martial Arts Federation National Fighters' Title Champions Trophy at Cartertons Sports Centre, Oxford at the weekend.

Paddy's triumph took his total of martial arts boxing official title records to seven, beating some of the country's top martial arts fighters.

He won his first three fights at the quarters and semi-final stage, and then had to fight five more challengers before reaching the finals.

He then won seven of his eight fights to claim the title, the winner being the man who won the most fights against his final rivals.

■ Paddy: Title king

His only defeat came in his fifth fight when a tired Paddy lost by just two points to an extremely sharp and fast Martyn Hobley of Broadwell, 101-99.

In the rest of the fights, Paddy's superior fitness and experience pulled him through against some very strong martial arts fighters.

Paddy has now achieved a world record of 1,956 competitive boxing and martial arts sparring rounds, and becomes the first ever registered martial arts instructor and former boxer to do so.

He is now going to concentrate on going for a black belt 4th dan and is preparing for his next fitness endurance record, which will be press-ups, to be attempted at Fairfield Air Show in July.

If successful, it will be his 98th feat. To date Paddy holds 97 National, European and World fitness endurance records.

The Observer, Thursday November 20, 2008

Strongman claims more records

BALSALL Common strongman Paddy Doyle signed off his 2008 season in style by claiming another two Guinness World Records - taking his tally for the year to 12.

A battleworn Paddy, who is still recovering from a slipped disc picked up at a strongman competition in America earlier this year, completed his final challenges for the season on Guinnes World Record Day (Thursday, November 13).

Setting off from Henley in Arden in the pouring rain, and with a 40lb backpack for company, tough guy Paddy broke two world records during a 30-mile mud-laden trek of the Arden Way which takes in Henley, Wootton Wawen, Aston Gantlow, Great Alne and Claverdon to name a few.

Despite the terrible conditions, Paddy claimed two new records - taking his career total to 166 of which he currently holds 75.

The first was for a 10km speed march carrying a 40lb backpack for which Paddy set a new record of 57minutes and two seconds - narrowly taking the title away from Rob Simpeon from Leeds who held it at 57minutes and 31 seconds.

The second was a new record for a winter speed march of the Arden Way, which the glutton for punishment completed in seven hours and 52 minutes.

"I'm chuffed to bits that I managed to get these records, but it was a tough day all round, mostly because of the horrible weather and the fact the route was so muddy," said Paddy.

"That's it for me for the year now though - I'm feeling a bit run down and battered and am going to give my body a rest over Christmas before looking at what records I can break next year."

Walk this way - Paddy Doyle during his latest record breaking attempt.
47.08.001.ab

The Gazette, Wednesday January 17, 2007

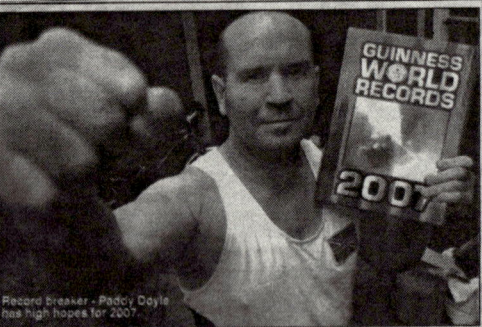

Record breaker - Paddy Doyle has high hopes for 2007.

Strongman bids to break more records

BALSALL Common strongman Paddy Doyle is gearing up to make 2007 his best year yet as part of a New Year resolution to break 20 world fitness records.

Paddy hasn't got any plans to put his feet up this year and is already training four hours a day to get his body ready for his toughest challenge to date.

The 20 records he intends to smash are currently held by rival American endurance athletes, including a 26-mile cross-country event carrying a 40 and 50lb back pack and various circuit training records.

At present Paddy currently holds 142 fitness endurance records recognised by four of the World Record Authorities.

As a result of his outstanding success in the world of physical endurance he has also been selected for a special United Kingdom vs America Fitness Endurance event in April, which will take place in both London and Coney Island in New York.

He is one of the 15 Brits who have been specially selected to take on American athletes to win the world physical endurance crown.

Paddy, a tutor at Solihull College said, he was stepping up his already punishing fitness regime.

"I vary the kind of exercise I do throughout the week and it ranges from boxing and martial arts to circuit training. "I have a great deal of support from my sports therapist on the kind of training I do and my diet.

"Ever since meeting my girlfriend, who is a vegetarian, I have substituted a lot of the meat I used to eat for vegetables and it's improved my performance both mentally and physically."

GERMAN CHALLENGE

I was invited to represent Great Britain once again at the World Record Games in Starnberg, Germany. The year was 2004. I had decided to attempt two World Fitness Endurance Records, the first being the World Ultra Fitness Record which consisted of eleven events. My training was tough and demanding. I was putting in three to four hours per day, sometimes getting home at 11.30pm. I would train in split shifts; for example, training for an hour and a half in the mornings and sometimes two to three hours after work. To be honest, my training diet was spread throughout the day. Due to work, my eating habits were erratic. However, I had to get on with the training and just get stuck in. What was uppermost in my mind was representing my country at the World Record Games. The officials from Germany contacted me and asked if I could attempt the World Cross Training Speed Record. I looked at the list and thought I could do that, although I had only one month to train for it. The challenge record is as follows:

- 1,750 metre swim
- 2,326 metres carrying 40lb back pack
- 20km run
- 10,000 metres rowing

- 20 mile cycle
- 3km stepper
- 2,000 star jumps
- 500 alternate squat thrusts
- 2,000 sit-ups
- weightlifting: 141 x 150kg lifted
- 1,400 machine hip flexors, 5kg attached

When I arrived at the venue I was told by the officials that I was to start the World Record at 10pm in the evening. Obviously I was pissed off by that, and fuming. My team members were Wayne Ferguson and Nigel Perry, and without their loyal support I do not think I would have achieved the World Record. Okay, I have attempted tougher fitness endurance challenges; however I had to take into account that I had arrived earlier in the day by plane, and made my own way from the airport to the venue the same evening, having had no rest or proper food.

Thank God I was experienced and focused on the attempt. 10pm came; the officials counted me down and I started the first physical fitness challenge which was the back pack run. As each mile, repetition and weight was recorded I was feeling very hungry. World Record team member Nigel Perry asked one of the German officials for some food, and I was brought boiled rice and salad which was ideal… at first. However, as I pushed my body further I needed a larger variety of food supplies. I asked the German officials for some more food and I was brought more rice and salad. I turned to Wayne Ferguson and said, 'More fuckin rabbit food.'

Wayne turned to the official, asking why the same food. He replied that all the officials were Vegans. I overheard what he said and went berserk. Wayne asked if there was a McDonalds nearby. He was directed to the local take-away, from which he brought me back a Big Mac.

I went non-stop throughout the night and finished the World Record at 11.59 the next morning. I collapsed and closed my eyes for a short time and I was then asked by the officials if I wanted to attempt the Guinness World Record for the most full contact kicks in one hour. The previous record, held by an American martial artist, stood at 1,085 kicks in one hour. I accepted and was dragged to my feet by Wayne and Nigel. My team members took it in turn to hold the pads. The counters were appointed German adjudicators. I have to admit I was feeling exhausted having just completed the fitness record throughout the night, but I carried on and broke the World Record with a total of 2,805 kicks in one hour.

'Thank fuck for that,' I said to Nigel, mighty relieved and exhausted. I was awarded two official diplomas and a trophy. We made our way back to the guest house and had a meal and a couple of bottles of red wine. The next morning we were back to the airport and later arrived safe and well at Birmingham airport. From the guest house to the airport I remember my joints and muscles aching all over; the whole of my body felt like a cardboard box. My joints were so stiff that every move I made took a few seconds longer than normal.

Only recently, I have found out that an American athlete has broken the World Record for the most full contact kicks in one hour. The new record is over 5,000, but he never achieved a 13-hour tough fitness endurance record as a warm-up, so if he thinks he beat me fair and square, he can think again.

The following Friday, Wayne and I went out to celebrate what I had achieved. We had a few beers and ended up in a curry house in Solihull. When we walked into the restaurant it was full with couples, and as time went by I noticed it was getting quieter. As I looked around the restaurant there were two blokes shouting and swearing at staff. They made eye contact with me and I heard one of them say, 'What the fuck's he looking at?'

I said nothing to Wayne, but just continued eating my curry. These two trouble makers had finished their meal and made their way to the door, where they sat for some time, looking at me. I decided to go to the bar which was situated near these two men. I knew they were waiting for me so I decided to make the first move. I swung around and hit one of them on the jaw. He landed on the floor. I hit the other on the side of his head and then chucked them both out through the door.

The waiters and manager watched in disbelief, a bit shocked at what they'd seen. Wayne sat there with his eyes wide open, also in disbelief. I have to thank him though; he got me out of the restaurant and in a taxi. The waiters and manager were totally on my side. They said the two loud-mouths had caused trouble before and, in their opinion, were intimidating the customers and me. Served themselves right, then. All the same, I was glad of my loyal pal, Wayne.

MOST DEMANDING WORLD RECORDS

I have always said that all of my fitness endurance, boxing, and martial arts titles and records have been tough, but there are a few which stand out from the rest. They are:

The most press-ups in 24 hours and most press-ups in a calendar year;

World United Martial Arts Association Warlords Kumite Title;

Endurance non-stop walk carrying a 9lb weight and 20lb back pack;

Guinness World Records Fittest Athlete Physical Fitness Challenge.

I will start off with the 24 hours press-up record. The previous at that time was 33,000 press-ups in 24 hours. I trained for eight months and the training sessions consisted of 10-mile runs, light weights, full contact boxing sparring and circuit training. The duration of the strict workouts was three to four hours, six days a week.

On some occasions I trained for twelve hours, doing press-ups, being helped by my loyal and close family friend, Desi Clifton, who patiently sat there counting and documenting each repetition and passing me water and fruit. The preparation was hard and demanding. My social life was non-existent. I went to bed some evenings at 9pm, rising at 5am the next morning to go for my early run. My breakfast consisted of liver tablets, cod liver oil, porridge oats, Ready Brek and wholemeal bread with fruit.

I could not wait for the day to come to attempt the World Record, but finally it came. I remember Desi Clifton saying to me, 'It is all up to you now, Paddy. You have to show you're the best in the world.'

I have to admit I was so nervous I was shitting myself. The main appointed senior official was then the World Masters Power lifting Champion, Ralph Farquharson. Ralph was a respected, genuine World Champion and judge in the World of power lifting. He briefed me on the Guinness World Records rules and regulations. I remember just nodding my head and staying focused, thinking about the next 24 hours. I was then shown to my changing room where I changed into my kit and discussed tactics with my training team.

An hour before the start, one of the officials came in to the room and said, 'Paddy, I am afraid to say I have some bad news.'

Bad news was not what I needed at that moment. The official said an athlete from Hong Kong had broken the Press-up World Record again in the early hours of that morning.

From that moment on, the new World Record was 35,000 press-ups. The news hit me like a bombshell, I realised I had to step up to the wire and push my body to the limits. Finally the midday start came and I was given the countdown to begin. I had to complete around 1,550 press-ups per hour with only a 5-minute rest break at the end of every hour.

Twelve hours into the record I was starting to feel mentally tired. My eyes were closing. Wayne Bernstein, one of the team members, marched me off to the toilets and got me to soak my head in cold water. This certainly woke me up and after a few minutes break and some bananas and apples, I continued to push myself. When 6am came I was doing press-ups with my eyes closed.

As the deadline approached, more spectators began to appear, which certainly kept me awake and made me more determined to break the World Record. In the last half-hour the noise was electrifying, gradually reaching fever pitch. Everyone was shouting. The officials announced, 'Paddy, you have one minute left.' I gave it my best shot and finished on time. Ralph Farquharson read out the total to the press and spectators.

'Ladies and gentleman, the new World Record is now… 37,350!'

I collapsed on the ground and my team picked me up. I gave a brief interview to the media and went to my hotel room. The officials and Desi Clifton came to my room to congratulate me, we had a drink and then all I remember was closing my eyes and sleeping for twenty-four hours. I could not move my body for about seven days. My joints and muscles ached, but it was worth every ounce of blood, sweat, pure grit and tears.

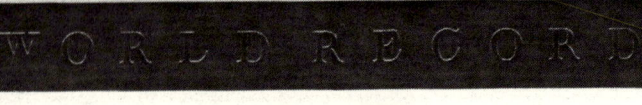

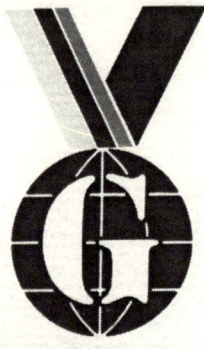

GUINNESS BOOK OF RECORDS

THIS IS TO CERTIFY THAT

PADDY DOYLE

PRESS UPS - 24 HOURS

37,350

HOLIDAY INN HOTEL

BIRMINGHAM

1-2 MAY 1989

DONALD McFARLAN   NORRIS McWHIRTER

The same year I was attempting the most press-ups in a calendar year. The previous record was held by Adam Parsons (USA). The date he completed the yearly record was 1984/85, his total being 1,293,850 press-ups.

The planning was the most difficult of all, I had to travel around the UK and complete 4,000 press-ups per day. The rules stipulated that I had to attempt the record at as many sporting venues as possible. Desi Clifton, John McBean and Billy Lawrence assisted me at most of the venues, their support being invaluable. On some occasions the officials did not turn up, which meant I had to do 8,000 press-ups the next day.

Once again my social life went out of the window for a whole year. I was focused on beating the World Record. My mates would ask me if I wanted to go out to a club or bar, but I had to refuse as I was hungry to be the Ultimate World Press-up Champion. The yearly press-up record supersedes all other press-up records and I wanted it badly.

The final day came. I had to complete 4,000 press ups to take the World Title. The spectators were again raising the roof with their encouragement. The countdown to complete the repetitions finally came. At last I had beaten the World Record. The new total was 1,500,250 press-ups. My eyes filled with tears and I heard a sigh of relief from Desi, John and Billy. I knew they were probably thinking, 'Thank fuck he has achieved it.'

I was awarded an official trophy and afterwards we cracked a few bottles of champagne with some food and started talking about the next challenge. I did not train for two weeks after the challenge. Rest was what my body needed and I remember thinking no more liquid cod liver oil and those dreaded liver tablets which looked like house bricks.

I have held that official World Record since 1989; no one has ever broken it since. As I have mentioned in previous interviews, I found that the documentation proving each daily total of press-ups was a challenge in itself. To claim a sports specific World Record you have to have the following paperwork for it to be approved: press cuttings, action photographs, DVD/Video footage, signed witness statements and signed judge/referee statements. If the paperwork does not meet the requirements the World Record could fail the approval process from the awarding body.

Ralf Laue, Editor of *The Book of Alternative Records 2009*, had this to say:

'Paddy Doyle's record for doing one and half million press-ups in one year is one of my all-time favourites listed in the *Book of Alternative Records*. It has been unbroken for twenty years. Paddy has never chosen the easy way. Just breaking a record is not what he is really interested in. The true challenge is to conquer and be the best in the World. I had the opportunity to witness two of Paddy's World Records in Germany. I think, on those occasions, I realised what really makes him tick. It is not just strength; it is not only pushing himself in the gym. It is mental power and discipline. All of us can learn a lot from him.'

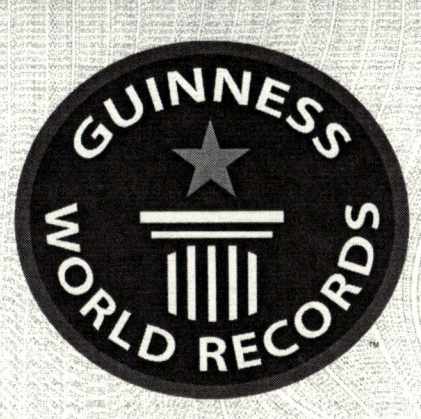

CERTIFICATE

The most push-ups performed (and documented) in one year is 1,500,230 by Paddy Doyle (GB) from 21 October 1988 to 21 October 1989

GUINNESS WORLD RECORDS LTD

Another category I have found ultra tough was the full contact karate boxing Kumite title record. Once you have a reputation, your opponents turn up for one reason only, to knock you out. Since 1993 I have won eleven full contact Kumite karate boxing grappling title records. These challenges consisted of fighting different registered/competitive fighters in every round. The rules were that I had to have a different opponent in each round. One minute I would be fighting a boxer, the next a black belt karate fighter. Two of my hardest opponents were Winston 'Spider' Harris (former seven times British Kickboxing Champion) and Carl Gibbs (former national heavyweight karate champion). These champions came to fight, not lie down.

The first time I fought Spider Harris was on the 21st August 1995. It was an experience and I soon found out why they nicknamed him Spider. His legs were everywhere. He was kicking me to the legs then switching his fast kicks to my head. During one exchange of blows I caught him with a left hook to the head which made him stumble. From experience he covered up and held on to me, which allowed him time to recover. The referee intervened and made us split from each other, by which time Spider Harris came back with a left kick to my head. I felt as though someone had sliced me with a knife.

Finally, the fight was over and the referee gave me the decision. In total I fought four fighters at the finale of the Kumite Title, achieving a total of 560 full contact karate boxing rounds in a calendar month.

The first time I fought Carl Gibbs was when I was attempting to win the World United Martial Arts

UK Kumite Open Weight Title Record, on 1st June 1997. The Kumite challenge was to fight the most full contact karate boxing rounds in ten days. The rules were the same as all the kumite challenge records I had fought. I had to fight different fighters in every round, all of whom were at black belt level. Carl Gibbs represented his club which was Corner Stone Karate Club in Sheldon, Birmingham. Heavyweight Gibbs was fast and furious. He was four stones heavier than I was, so I had to move quickly and throw fast left and rights to his head and body.

His straight left punch was powerful; it caught me a few times to the jaw and body. I knew if I used my speed and power I would win the rounds. At last the referee, Ronnie Christopher (twenty seven times Karate National, European and World Champion) shouted time. The contest was awarded to me but I have to admit it was close. I had thrown some powerful punches thinking I would have worn him down, but the mighty Gibbs took them well and kept coming forward. For that title record, I fought five martial artists and boxers. The finishing total of competitive full contact rounds fought in ten days against other fighters who came to Stamina's Gym to fight me was 251. The final results of the challenge were as follows:

Neil Gray (light heavy) v Paddy Doyle (middleweight) I won on points.
Peter Shephard (super middleweight) v Paddy Doyle. I won on points.
Vince Brotherton (light middleweight) v Paddy Doyle. I won on points.

Carl Gibbs (Heavyweight) v Paddy Doyle. I won on points.
Winston 'Spider' Harris v Paddy Doyle. Match drawn.

Another memorable moment was when I set a new kumite karate boxing record for the most full contact rounds in a calendar month. The date for the final was 21 August 1995. The reason I have never forgotten this challenge was because I was still carrying injuries from a World Record I achieved ten days earlier. That fitness record was for the most squat thrusts in two hours. My feet had blisters which were starting to burst, and my ankles and knees were stiff. I knew that mentally I had to cut the mustard and forget about the pain. Mark Richards, the local sports reporter for the *Heartland Evening News*, based in Nuneaton, was in the crowd and reporting on the Title Record. His report is as follows:

Mark Richards, Sports Reporter, Evening Heartland News, 24 Aug 1995.
'By now everyone must have heard about the weekend's boxing match between Mike Tyson and Peter McNeeley, that turned out to be 89 seconds work. That said, and referring to someone much closer to home, what sum would you give a boxer for 560 rounds of what can only be described as thrilling – Rocky Balboa style – action? I'm a fan of boxing and also a realist. So when I'm asked to go along to a fight where one man will take on four, I'll be honest, I laughed so much, I just had to go and watch for myself, just to see that man lose.

Let's face it, no one in their right mind would back anything when the odds are four to one, over 12 rounds, one of which included three boxers at once. But what if that man just happened to be record-breaking Paddy Doyle? Would you think again? Still no? Then read on. Yes, like everything else this popular Brummie does, this challenge was about breaking yet another World martial arts record, his 77th to be exact. The challenge? To achieve the most rounds of boxing and karate in one calendar month. His target to beat was 538, his personal task being more than 20 rounds a day for 28 days. To spar, as defined in the Collins dictionary, means 'to box using light blows as in training.'

Well why didn't anyone tell Paddy or his opponents that? If they had, then a lot of pain and grief would have been spared. The Holly Lane Sports and Social Club was the scene for Paddy's latest attempt. A far cry from Tyson's magnificent MGM Grand Hotel in Las Vegas. The seating was the odd stool if you could find one, the 'ring' was ten mats pushed together and the air conditioning was a couple of broken windows. With the odds totally stacked against him on Monday night, and even though the record was already, mathematically, in the bag, Paddy faced his four foes: Winston 'Spider' Harris, a British kick boxing champion; Glyn Davis; Ian Parkes, a former army boxer, and the tall, awkward heavyweight, Neil Grey.

Spider was the first up and, just like a Bruce Lee film, came out kicking and punching. Using his experience, Paddy closed ranks and as the crowd started to hiss, he erupted. Eyes wide with rage, he unleashed a flurry of right and lefts. If you blinked, then you missed it. Round one and Harris was on the canvas. Totally bewildered with the assault he'd just taken, Spider's pride forced him to carry on. The Ref looked into his eyes; with a glimmer of hope staring back at him, he gave the clearance. Holding back, Paddy allowed Harris to come to his senses and, before he knew it, time was called.

Up came number two. Tough Glyn Davis was his name, and he towered above the Midlands hero. As with the first round, Paddy faced a fighter who wanted to rock the apple cart. The punches were fast and furious. Paddy closed ranks again, played the waiting game, and unleashed another terrific combination which had Davis on his backside. Time was up, and then in came number three, Ian Parkes. Another case of déjà vu, Parkes coming out all guns blazing and being outboxed. The fifth and most interesting of all rounds was complete and utter madness. Three fighters in three minutes and, you've guessed it, there was only one victor. Paddy Doyle.

It looked like a bar room brawl of the highest quality. This was skill, determination and dedication only possessed by professional athletes. The four against Paddy soon became eight and then twelve, as fellow fighters who arrived late, advised those up against it 'how to get him.' By the eighth round, the crowd had swelled, and the fighters had clearly lost the battle, but determinedly soldiered on against the former paratrooper.

I had to ask the question. 'Just what was it like facing Paddy?'

Spider, still panting from his beating, spluttered,

'He's an animal… an animal. I don't know how he does it, but he still keeps coming at you.'

I pitched the next question: 'What's your next plan to beat him?'

The fighters replied as one. 'We need to have a go together and take the big one with us.' The 'big one' referred to was reigning world heavyweight kickboxing champion, Pele Reid.

Pele chipped in, 'Paddy defies everything. He's small, yeah, but he throws a punch like a heavyweight. I should know, because I've taken them.

The object of the evening, just like this piece, wasn't to show what this one-man army could do, although I do admit it must read like that. But, no, it was to see the man, who is on a life long mission to capture the ultimate record crown for the most strength speed stamina records ever held by one man. Okay, I must have lost count how many times I have spoken to Paddy and seen his celebratory picture in the press after a world record. But I had never seen him in action, and believe me, I wouldn't have missed this for the world.

Paddy's payment for the 560 rounds was 100,800 seconds, a foot-high trophy to show he captured the World United Martial Arts Association full contact Kumite Record, and a certificate… all accepted with a big, broad smile.'

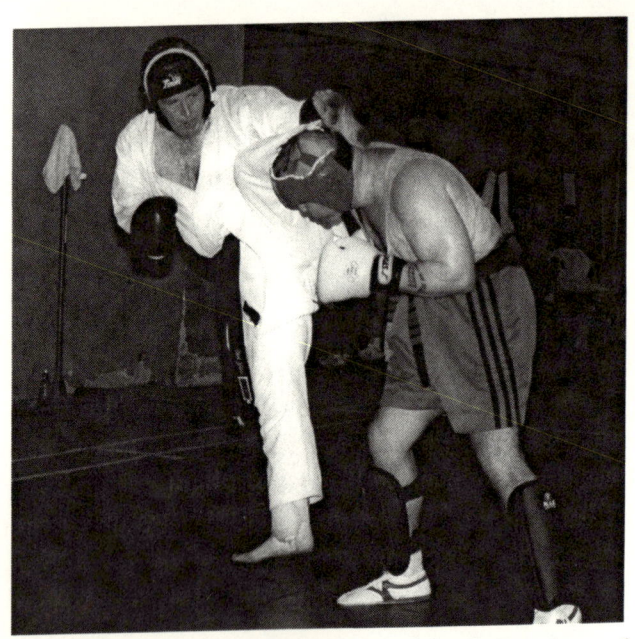

{Carl Gibbs "heavyweight" verse Paddy Doyle in the WUMA Kumite Challenge Title Record Challenge. 9 June 2002}

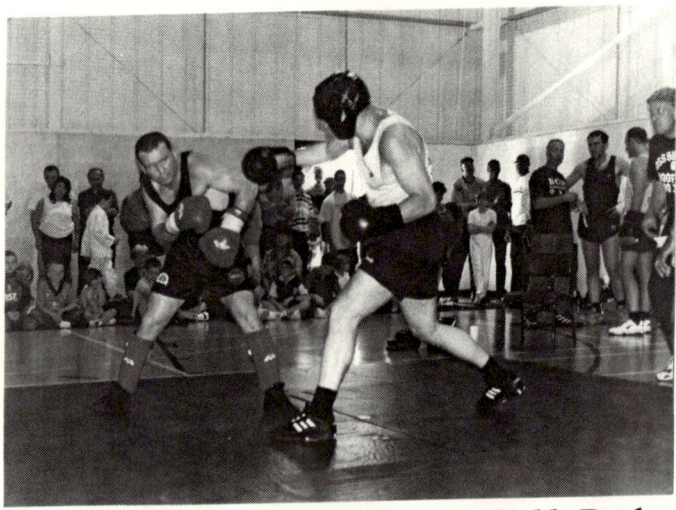

{Neil Grey "light heavy weight" verse Paddy Doyle. 1 June 1997}

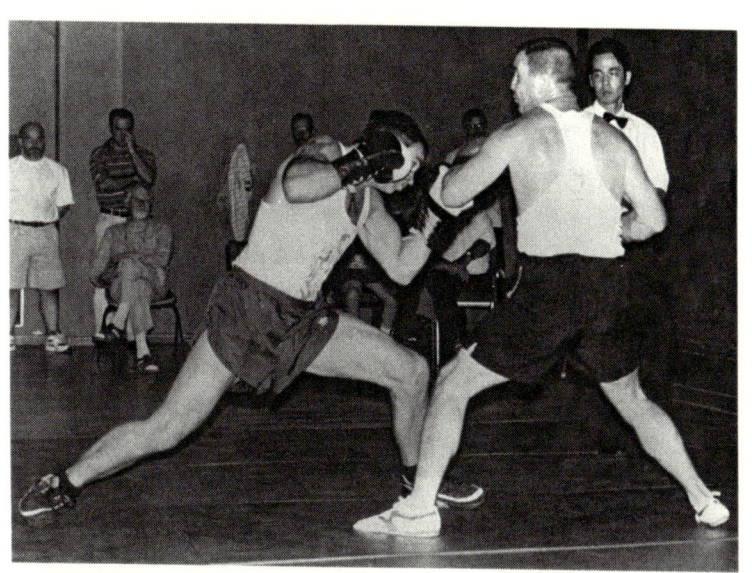

{Ian Parkinson Verse Paddy Doyle "won on points" WUMA Kumite Full Contact Karate - Boxing Title Record. 23 September 1996}

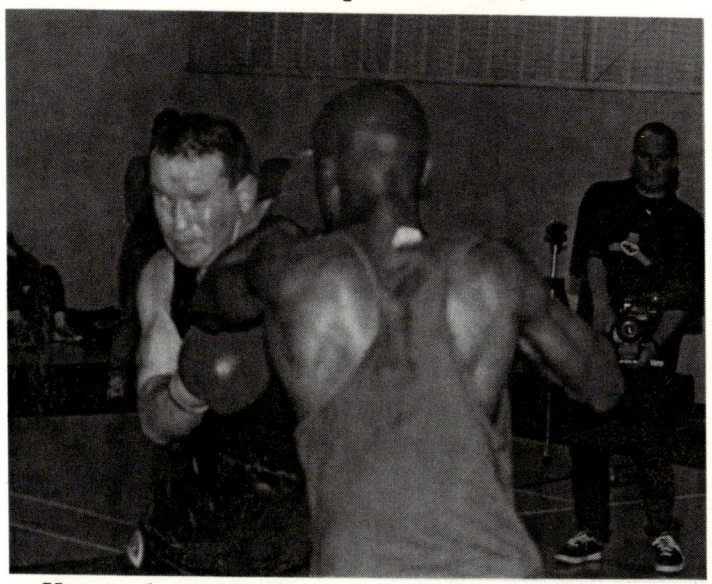

Kumite karate boxing rounds. {Most Fullcontact karate boxing rounds in one month, total 560}

The speed press-ups records have also been hard to break. When I started my endurance athletic career, the first speed record I went for was the most push-ups in 37 minutes. I know what you are thinking and agree with you that 37 minutes is an odd number, but there was a record to beat which was held by Masura Noma of Japan. His record total was 1,227 push ups. And the second record I set was the most push ups in 3hrs 54mins. For these records I had to drop my weight by 8lbs. The secret was to have a light body weight, otherwise you could not maintain the amount of repetitions you had to knock out to beat the records.

I beat one and set a new European record on 25 February 1989 at Le Pub in Birmingham City Centre. A large crowd turned out to see if I could smash two records in one day. All I can remember is the lactic acid burning, but once again my first loyal training coach, Desi Clifton (a former Karate Instructor and fighter) and my pacers just kept me going to the end. Everything was a blur. All I can remember is starting and finishing and the officials shaking my hand.

I suppose I was starting to realise what goal-setting meant and how strong my mind was. From that day onwards I went from strength to strength. I beat the Japanese record of 1,740 push ups in 37mins, and set a new European record of 7,860 push ups on the same day. My team and Desi went to celebrate at another local pub… and guess what? We got a little pissed.

The Guinness Record for the most miles walked carrying a 10 lb concrete slab / brick in a nominated hand, in a downward position, pushed me mentally. The pain at some stages of the attempt was unbearable.

Although I have attempted this challenge twice before, I knew when I attempted it for the third time, what I was up against. Plus it was not going to be any easier. My team and I decided to go for the record again. The other main reason was to raise vital funds for brothers Thomas and Samuel Deakin. Samuel aged 11 yrs has a life threatening brain tumour, and Thomas aged 5 has cerebral palsy. Money raised from the record will go towards a well earned holiday for the family who have been through a tough time. The date was set 21 May 2009. The current record I had to beat was 78 mile. 7121 yards, held by Suresh Joachim {Sri Lanka}.

The team and I set off at 2.30am, the reason for starting earlier was because it was cooler, and the weather forecast for the rest of the day said that the temperature would rise. The officials and pacers were at check point number one and ready to go. Alan Deakin karate Instructor , Terry Carruthers Professional boxer and Andy Collins were the first to escort and pace me around the course route. My greatest worry at this point was falling and injuring my ankle, but we all had torches and the appropriate kit to deal with any accidents. As the day went by my arm, wrist, shoulder and lower back were giving me a lot of pain and cramp, but the pacers kept me going by talking to me which took my mind off the physical discomfort.

The second batch of pacers took over. At this stage my feet were covered in blisters. Some of them had burst which had made my feet stick to my socks, and inner soles of my boots. Paul Jones martial arts instructor,

Colin Dickinson official, Stewart Mitchinson West Mercia Police Detective Sergeant, and Jamie McGuire had the responsibility of keeping me going and staying focused. The temperature had risen at this stage.

My head was lowering and I started to get grumpy with myself, but I knew the record was in the bag. All I had to do was dig deep putting my mind on a goal setting level. Each checkpoint near the end seemed to be lasting forever. My legs were feeling weak due to the heat and carrying the weight. When I reached every checkpoint Brian Vernum the checkpoint official, would pass me a hot drink and some food which gave me much needed energy to keep walking.

Students from the Corner Stone Karate Club joined the walk for the last 9 mile, this was a massive boost for me, as I was weak mentally and physically. As the miles were adding up I could see the light at the end of the tunnel. The official shouted out to the pacers and walkers "Paddy has only half a mile to go!" It was a great feeling to see the finish line so we all picked up the pace and finally I reached checkpoint one. The official informed the walkers and team that I had walked carrying a 10 lb brick in a nomitted hand and a 15 lb back pack, a distance of 80.372 miles beating the previous Guinness World Record by over a mile. I then thanked everyone for their support. It is hard to explain how I felt. I was mentally fatigued and my whole body was shaking, plus the power in my right hand and arm had gone. My body was smelling of sweat and the top of my head was red raw from the sun. I was pleased with my performance as I had minimal injurys, I slept for two days solid.

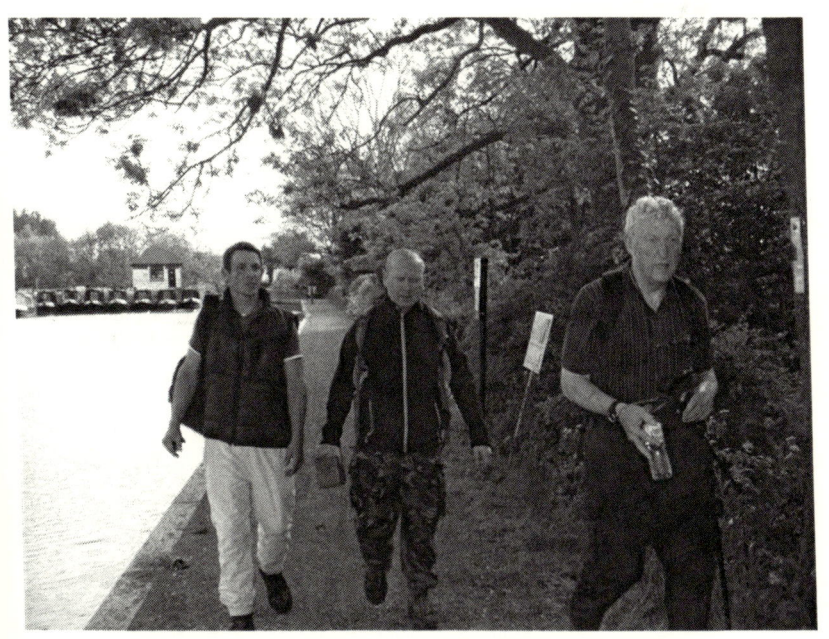

{World Record - Most miles walked carrying a 10 lb concrete slab / brick with smooth sides, in a downward pinch grip position, total distance 80.372 miles. Broken on 21 May 2009 UK.}

World's Fittest Athlete Physical Fitness Challenge Record

This is the toughest cross training World Record and I am proud of it. I trained solidly for eight months to build up my strength, speed and stamina. The previous World Title was held by an American athlete who set an impressive overall time of 19hrs 21mins. My training consisted of running up to 10 miles daily, 1-2 miles of swimming, weightlifting, circuit training, rowing up to 15 miles, 10-15 miles on the cross trainer and 40-50 miles cycling. My training programme would be split into different sections. For example, I would never row every day. I would have variations, concentrating on different parts of my body.

To prepare for this World Title your body and mind must be finely tuned. As part of the preparation, I would train every Thursday at the martial arts boxing club with my students. The training involved full contact sparring, circuit training, shadow boxing, bag work and light weights. I clearly remember to this day how lonely I felt. I had to shut myself off from socialising with my friends, and think solely about the challenge that lay ahead. I had to eat, sleep and focus on training if I were to be the first Briton to hold the ultimate World Record for all-round fitness.

Finally the big day came. I was nervous. What if I sustained an injury in the first few hours? My team and the appointed officials started to arrive. I was briefed on the rules and regulations and then told to warm up and get ready for the countdown. At last I was given the go ahead and started the first event which was the 12-mile run.

As each event was successfully completed throughout the day, my mind was in a trance as though I were looking down a long tunnel. The last four hours were a struggle. I was starting to lose concentration and felt tired. Cramp started to set in and I honestly thought I was not going to make that one. But the spectators arriving at the Gym got behind me, shouting non-stop. The support was unbelievable.

Finally, I came to the last exercise challenge. I had to complete 1,250 push-ups. My arms were in pain from the weightlifting. Once again my mind started to wander. I wanted to curl up and sleep there and then…

All of a sudden, the team members were shouting down my ear, 'Get your fuckin' arse moving, Doyle, otherwise you won't beat the World Record!'

My mind kicked in again and I knew there were only thirty minutes to go for the final countdown. When the official in charge of the stop watch said five minutes to go, I just battled my way to the finish, forcing out as many push-ups as possible. The next time I heard his voice, he was saying, 'Thirty seconds to go…' Tears were streaming down my face. My mind and body were near to collapse. A loud voice shouted time. The torture was finally over and, above the cheering, one of the judges read out what I had completed, along with the time.

'In 18 hours 56 minutes and 9 seconds, Paddy Doyle, representing Great Britain completed the following physical fitness challenges:

12-mile run; 12-mile speed march walk (carrying a 25lb backpack); 1,250 star jumps; 3,250 sit-up crunches; 1,250 hip flexors (10lb weight); 110-mile cycle; 20-mile rowing; 20-mile gym cross trainer; weightlifting 300,000 lb various lifts; 2-mile swim and 1,250 push ups.'

I was then awarded an official World Record Certificate and a trophy by my former Sergeant Major, Eddie Barron from the Royal Fusiliers TA Regiment. I have to admit I was at breaking point. My joints started to seize up. I was tearful and for some unknown reason I felt the loneliest athlete in the World. A World Record challenge at that level does something to your brain; you are pushing the pain barrier to the extreme. I believe that Guinness World Records no longer requires athletes to complete the hip flexors lifting the 10lb weight, but at least I know I broke the World Record the hard way.

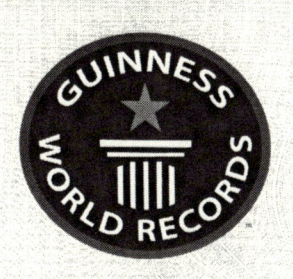

CERTIFICATE

The fastest time to complete the physical fitness challenge is 18 hr 56 min 9 sec achieved by Paddy Doyle (UK) at the Virgin Active health club, Solihull, UK, on 16 February 2005. The challenge consists of the following: 12 mile march, 12 mile speed march (25 lb pack), 1,250 push ups, 1,250 star jumps, 3,250 sit up crunches, 1,250 hip flexors (10 lb weight), 110 mile cycle, 20 mile row, 20 mile cross trainer, 2 mile swim, weightlifting lifted 300,000 lb upper body lifts only.

GUINNESS WORLD RECORDS LTD

Guinness Certificate {Guinness Physical Fitness Challenge Record Title 2005}

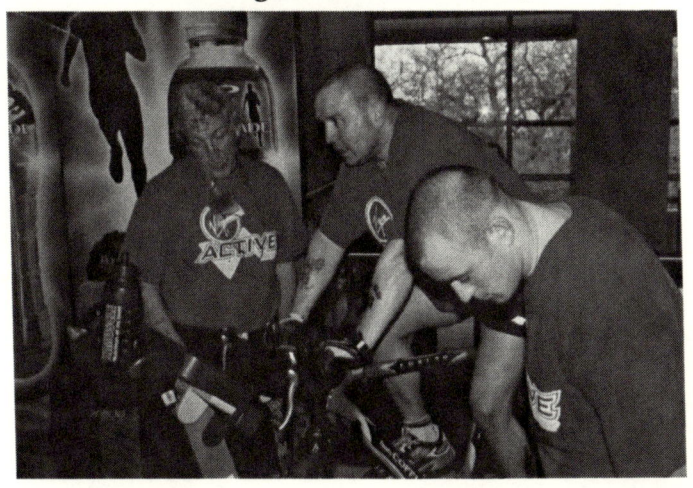

{Guinness Physical Fitness Challenge Record, 110 mile cycle event. 16th Feb 2005}

'Dean Gould, Editor of *Alternative Book of Records and Record Holders Association* (2007)** had this to say: 'Paddy's variation on all athletic records shows that he has a great mind. The one mile 40lb back pack record is the one I rate very highly, as you think of Bannister, Coe, Ovett and Cram, only they could not beat this incredible time. Paddy has all three things a person could wish for in life. Thousands of people have run marathons, but Doyle's title of the World's Fittest Athlete tops them all, as only a handful of World Record class athletes could even complete it. He happens to be the best. He has set some high benchmarks with all of his titles and records. But like any genuine World Record Holder he must always look back and think he could have done better. He need not worry as most of his sporting endurance records will still stand in fifty years' time.'

The endurance non-stop walk carrying a 9lb weight in a nominated hand with a 20lb back pack was a mentally tough record. The rules stated that I had to walk carrying a 9lb weight in a nominated hand in a locked position. The time was not recorded; only the distance was logged. This challenge was tiring because I had to carry the weight in an awkward position. My arm and hand were soon feeling like lead weights and my shoulder muscles were on fire.

The team who were supporting me were also feeling the pace. Colin Dickinson (appointed official) was the main lynch pin in organising the pacers and meeting us at certain check points along the Grand Union Canal. We made an early start at 5.30am from Birmingham

City Centre. Paul Jones walked with me for the first 20 miles along with other pacers. Although they were not carrying any weight they were feeling tired and wanted a rest. Every hour I was allowed a five-minute toilet and food break. Colin, his wife Wendy, and Paul made sure I got plenty of food down me. Without their insistence that I ate and drank I would never have been able to carry on with the World Record. When I reached the forty-mile mark, some of the team members were feeling tired and started to moan to each other about how tough it was getting. I believe Colin or Paul turned round to some of the pacers and reminded them that I was doing the record and not them.

The pacers realized that I was not moaning and that they were only pacing me for short distances. When I had been on my feet for twenty-five hours, my mind was elsewhere. I was starting to hallucinate and I was talking to myself. It was the only way to stay awake, otherwise I would not have broken the record. At last I was informed that I had only four miles to go. By then I could hardly stand and Paul and Colin walked either side of me, urging me to stay awake.

Finally, I reached the finishing line after twenty-eight hours without any sleep. The distance covered was 77 miles 350 yards, beating the previous record held by Jamie Borges (USA) of 73 miles. I collapsed on the ground, my body shaking all over. My eyes looked like piss-holes in the snow, the right side of my body cramped up, and the blisters on my feet were red raw and bleeding from the constant pounding. When I got home I stayed in bed for two whole days. My legs felt like iron bars; I had to crawl to the bathroom. But it was worth it; at the end of the day another record had bitten the dust. I can only thank the pacers and officials who stood by me and pushed me to achieve my goal.

Solihull Observer
SPORT

PAGE 25

Martial arts record for Paddy

The Observer, Thursday January 31, 2008

FITNESS guru Paddy Doyle smashed five martial art world records at a Birmingham gym last week.

The Balsall Common strongman pushed himself to new limits when he set the new records at Stamina's Gym in Erdington on Thursday, January 21.

Displayinig his usual stamina and endurance, Paddy completed 124,963 punch strikes in 12 hours, 29,850 punches in one hour; 7,668 punches in 15 minutes, 2,128 punches in five minutes and 702 punches in one minute.

In all five categories he took the titles from former champions including Angelo Breaux, Howard Smith and Roberto Ardito.

During the successful record breaking attempt Paddy endured torn bicep muscles, bruised knuckles and an upper back and neck injury. He has no plans to stop his world record breaking attempts.

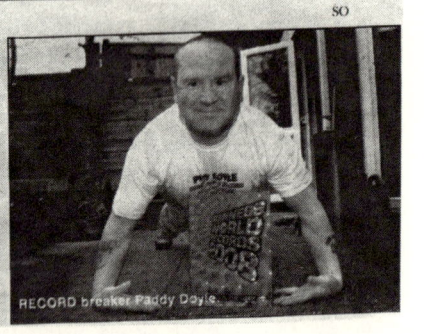

RECORD breaker Paddy Doyle.

MAGAZINE OF THE BRITISH ARMY
SOLDIER
NOVEMBER 2006 £2.50

Paddy power

PARATROOPER-turned-record-breaker Paddy Doyle notched up his 141st endurance record by capturing the World Ultra Fitness title at Gleasons Boxing Gym in Brooklyn.

Already recognised as the World's Fittest Athlete, the former Territorial Army fusilier secured his latest world record – his first on American soil – by completing a gruelling set of five one-hour physical challenges.

During the non-stop record attempt Doyle ran 5.05 miles carrying a 40lb bergen, completed 512 30-feet shuttle sprints with the 40lb bergen and cycled 21.6 miles.

The amateur boxer and mixed martial artist also completed 713 30lb standing chest presses and 835 step-ups, again with the 40lb load.

"This record proved particularly tough because I was in America on my own, without my support team," Doyle told *SoldierSport*.

"With temperatures topping 101F I really had to push my body to the limit, but although it was hard going I thoroughly enjoyed the challenge."

NOVEMBER 2006

SPORT
Friday July 20 2007

Sports editor: Simon Steele
Phone 01926 457730 Fax 339960
Email sport@leamingtoncourier.co.uk

Another world record for super-fit Doyle

PADDY Doyle successfully tackled a tough cross-country marathon to set his 148th fitness and endurance world record.

Former paratrooper Doyle, who lives in Balsall Common, donned a 45lb backpack to run up hills, wade through streams and climb stiles, completing the tough Arden Cross Country Marathon course in 7hr 37min 2sec - much faster than the 9.08.0 he managed in February while carrying a 40lb pack.

Although he suffered an ankle injury after 11 miles, the self-styled British bulldog dug deep and pushed himself to the finishing line, helped by his pacers and officials.

THURSDAY, JULY 5, 2007 Birmingham Mail 25

East City News
Match fit for challenge

SHELDON

SHELDON-born world fitness champion Paddy Doyle is setting his sights on adding another title to his ever-growing list.

Rain will fail to stop play on Saturday as Paddy powers through wind and high water on the gruelling 26-mile Arden Challenge through Warwickshire's countryside carrying a 40lb backpack.

The former paratrooper is hoping to clinch his 148th world record title by completing the trek in less than nine hours and eight minutes - a record he set in January.

"I know I could have done better so I'm going back to have another go," said Paddy, 42, who lives in Balsall Common.

"The weather in January was terrible and obviously those kinds of conditions make the going slower.

"I'm hoping for better weather on Saturday, but even if it's terrible the date's been arranged for a long time so it's too late to change it.

Paddy, who is officially the World's Fittest Athlete, said he was hoping to trounce his previous time and has been working hard to get ready for the feat.

"I'm really looking forward to the challenge," added Paddy, who runs the Access to the Military Course at Solihull College.

"I've been practising with a 65lb backpack so I'm more than ready for it."

41

HARD TIMES AND MAKING ENDS MEET

I came from a broken home. My mother left us when I was around three years of age. She went to live with another man, whom I ended up liking very much. My sister Bridget looked after me for a short while, but when she was sixteen she moved out and got a job and a flat elsewhere. My father then took over the reins and brought me up.

As time passed, he met a woman named Barbara, who took on the role of step-mother. I was a handful for her as I'd had no discipline. Prior to Barbara coming into my life, I used to be out until midnight at the age of six. I was either smashing factory windows or pinching sweets from the corner shop, or ringing doorbells and legging it as fast as I could, or throwing stones at buses.

When Barbara laid down the new rules, I was rebelling all the time. I could not adjust to the change. When I did play up, I sometimes got a hard slap around my head, and I remember that my ears use to ring for a couple of days afterwards. On other occasions when I was very cheeky and rude, she would lock me in my bedroom for hours. I would be left with a bucket to piss and poo in. My dinner would be brought to me between 5pm and 6pm. The door would be unlocked and she would put my dinner down on the floor. I would then be allowed to go to the toilet and empty the bucket. Back in the bedroom she would then lock the door again and I would eat my dinner. I could not open the window as she had screwed it down. She obviously thought I would have run away and she was right.

When my father came home from work, the door would be unlocked just before he came into the house. I was too scared to say anything to him about what had happened to me, because I thought that when he went back to work I would be punished and locked away again. So my dad, who was a kind and loving father, never knew what was going on. He probably thought everything was fine, but it never was. Let's face it… when you are between seven and nine years of age, how do you express yourself? At that age, I thought that all my mates were being treated the same. Although Barbara was trying to do her best and taking on the role of my mother, it was just not working.

I was allowed to see my mother every Sunday for four hours. This was agreed by the Court. So from the age of about six, I met my mom. But we always went to bingo halls. My mom, whom I loved very much, was hooked on bingo. Whilst she was occupied with trying to win the bloody jackpot, I was eating cheese sandwiches or feeding money she had given me into the fruit machines… one-armed bandits, we called them then. This carried on until I was fourteen. I then told Mom that I would pretend to meet her every Sunday and do my own thing with my mates. So every Sunday, my dad and Barbara mistakenly thought I was meeting my mother. When I became sixteen I left my dad and went to live with my mother.

It did hurt me to leave my dad, but I could not stand the rules Barbara was ordering me to abide by. I had no choice but to leave, as it was her house and not my father's. In May 2008 I discovered that Barbara had passed away. I was contacted by a nurse who had looked after her. She told me when the funeral was. It was the day after I had achieved four World Records. I remember when I got up the next morning I could not move due to the stiffness and injuries I had sustained.

Something made me go along to the funeral. What it was, I will never know. I mentioned to the nurse that I had dropped round to her house some months previously and left my contact card. The nurse told me that she had received it and, allegedly, had asked Barbara if she would like to see me. She told the nurse that she would have nothing to say to me. That said it all, really.

I still went to the funeral, but I felt numb, somehow, and rather put out. I thought to myself that I should not have bothered turning up. This is the first time I have voiced my feelings about this. All I remember when I lived with her was mental torture and being hit hard around the head.

My mom lived in a damp and cold bedsit in Kings Road, Erdington. There was no central heating and we had hardly any money. The walls were damp and in the winter months there was frost on the inside of the windows every morning. My mom and I would race to the kitchen, close the door and put the gas cooker on to warm the place up. I knew I had to bring some money in fast.

I managed to get a part-time job, working on a market stall in Birmingham City Centre. That only lasted for two days as I was caught stealing from my employer. So I decided to try other methods of bringing in supplies to keep us going. I got up at 5am and made my way to the corner shop. At this time of the morning the delivery trucks would drop off their stock and leave it outside the shop door. I timed it by my watch that it took around five to seven minutes for the shop owner to come downstairs and bring in the delivery.

I used to hide in the alleyway or the public park opposite until the delivery man had gone and then run over to the shop front and help myself to a selection of newspapers, sweets and a couple of bottles of milk. My method was to alternate from shop to shop. The corner shops were based on Brookvale Road and Slade Road, Erdington. I did not want to set a pattern stealing from the same shop every morning. If I did that I would certainly be caught. This carried on for a couple of weeks until one morning when I was waiting to steal the goodies, the shop owner was already waiting outside with a baseball bat. I carefully shrank back into the bushes and disappeared. That was the end of that. One thing that will always stay in mind was that my mother and I used to have a laugh about it. Well… that's life.

My mother finally got a council house in a suburb called Quinton, which is on the outskirts of Birmingham. The house was in Dufton road. It was a quiet road then, full of retired people. I then started boxing training at the Austin Amateur Boxing Club, and weightlifting at the Harborne Weightlifting Centre. I was training very hard six days a week, so I decided to get a job which would pay for my food and vitamin tablets.

I finally got a job at a food chain store based in Five Ways, Edgbaston just outside the City Centre. I was pushing trolleys and filling shelves. The money was rubbish but it was the only place that would take me on. I was there for about twelve months and whilst I was there, there were regular thefts from the store by professional shoplifters. The management and security staff were relying on me to help out and restrain the shoplifters until the Police arrived.

This was an excellent opportunity for me to build up a relationship with the Security team and Senior Managers. Once the trust was built up, I started robbing the store. The items I was taking were spirits and electrical goods which I would sell to acquaintances and members of the Gym. Some of the money would pay for my Gym fees and food, and the rest would go to my mother to pay the bills. Mom and I were still short of cash so I had to put my hand to anything to bring in the money to put food on the table.

That job came to an end as I fell out with some of the workers and managers. I was asked to leave by the store manager, Mr Williams. He said to me, 'Paddy, I like you, but you are intimidating and scaring some of the staff and managers. I'll tell you what I will do for you. I will give you four months pay and a good reference if you leave quietly.' I accepted and left.

Being involved in a minority sport means financial

support is hard to come by, so sometimes you have to take desperate measures. On one occasion a food manufacturer approached me to do some surveillance on his factory premises. Apparently one of the employees was stealing food from the main stores and selling it on to other food suppliers. So for four nights I carried out a surveillance on the building from 11pm to 6am. It also happened to be in the winter. Sometimes it would rain non-stop and other nights it would be bloody freezing.

Some nights, the rain would be pounding down on me as I hid in the bushes. The reason for me being outside was because the parcels were being taken from the factory and put into the vehicles. I had one lucky escape, when I got close to the employee who was suspected of taking the items. I was only a metre away in the bushes and he still could not see me. He appeared to be looking straight at me, but still could not see me, probably because I was camouflaged and kitted out correctly. Unfortunately, he never stole when I was watching him. The owner of the business was still concerned as he was still losing stock from his factory. I had a meeting with him and advised him that it would be better if I had two other men to help watch the premises from different angles.

The two men I was hoping would help me were ex-soldiers, but at the last minute they could not make it. I had to ring around to see if anyone else was available and ended up with Barmy Brian, who is a close friend. By coincidence, I had another friend, named Bryan, who was 73 and retired. Neither had any experience of night surveillance work, so I had to show them the basics very quickly. We arrived near the factory premises and walked in. I allocated both of them an area they could see from a camouflaged position.

We kept in contact by mobile phone and a walkie-talkie. At around 2am Barmy Brian came over the radio.

'Paddy, I think the old feller has fallen asleep. I can hear him snoring.'

I had to make my way around the wooded area and check if he was okay. Thankfully he was awake. I made my way back to my view point and carried on with the watch. At 3.30am I got another call from Barmy Brian.

'Paddy, I can hear noises behind me. I think someone is there.'

Once again I left my view point, and made my way directly to Barmy Brian.

'What's the problem, Brian?'

He was nervous. 'There's something in them fuckin' bushes, Paddy.'

I went to the place he was pointing to, moved the bushes and came face to face with a cow looking over the farm fence. It was turning into a comedy sketch and I was getting pissed off with running from one position to the next. The final outcome was that nothing was stolen that night. I remember that we could not stop laughing in the car on the way back home. Thank God the owners of the business did not know what went on, but it did make me some extra cash to pay for my food, supplements, and training kit.

On another occasion, a businessman who owned a betting shop approached me. He wanted me to sort out a former business partner who was harassing him and had been smashing up his car and house for three years. We had an in-depth conversation during which I gave him a price for my services. We agreed a deal and I was given the bloke's address and telephone number and the name of his local.

I managed to trace his whereabouts, spoke to him in a very polite manner and, to my surprise, he suddenly stopped harassing the businessman. But the bully wanted to get me back another way for pulling him. He knew he could not beat me physically so he approached some blokes to sort me out. As it happened, the heavies he approached knew me. 'We're not fuckin' with him,' they said, and stayed out of it. Since then the businessman and I have become friends and he has supported me financially in achieving some of my sporting goals.

When I lived in Sheldon, a suburb of Birmingham, there was a local grocery I used on a regular basis. All the items were labelled with a price tab. On many occasions I would go into the shop and swap over the price tabs to a reduced price. This helped my shopping bill and saved me a lot of money. My reason for doing this was because I was short of money, and needed food to train. Sometimes the owner, whom I have now got to know very well, would look at me suspiciously. I think he knew what I was up to but he let me get away with it, because he probably felt sorry for me.

There was one year – 2000 – when I found it very hard to get any support from sports companies or Birmingham-based businesses. That year was also difficult for me as I was short of cash. I was dismissed from my job for threatening the management and also for taking time off to train for a World Record. I suppose it was my own fault. I was going through a bad time with a relationship, so I decided to go sick for about six weeks. I was later called into work and asked why I had been off sick when one of the managers had seen my name in the local paper, winning the World United Martial Arts Karate Boxing Kumite Title. I had fought 131 contact rounds against different black belts in 5 hours at the WUMA HQ, Cheltenham in May. I had no answer and I was shown the door. I did feel let down by my coordinator at that time, who set me up. Another manager who attended the disciplinary hearing confirmed this to me. He, and indeed other senior managers, thought he had backstabbed me. Although I was in the wrong, I should not have placed my trust in the coordinator.

But I got the two-faced bastard back in more ways than one. I have learnt from experience that giving someone a good hiding does not always work, as they always call the law. So you get them back mentally. When they go to bed at night it plays on their mind and can affect their daily working life. Another manager based at the same Educational Centre was pissing me off. His position then was the marketing manager. One morning I asked him if he wanted a cup of coffee. He thanked me for my kindness. As it happened, the toilets were just down the corridor and I rushed straight to them, pretending I was going to clean the cups. When the toilets were clear, I pissed, spat and put an Exlax tablet in the cup. One tablet would give you diarrhoea for a week. I then added coffee and sugar and topped it up with hot water. Then I watched him drink it whilst we discussed work issues. I later found out that he'd had to go home early that afternoon... he felt sick with stomach cramps. Served the back-stabbing asshole right, I thought.

A contact of mine rang me to say he had some trainers in stock and could I sell some for him. I told him how much I wanted per pair if I sold any, and he agreed. I thought he was only talking about four or five pairs of trainers but when he came round to my house he dropped off one hundred pairs in four large boxes. I stood in my lounge wondering how the fuck was I going to sell that lot?

I got on the phone straight away, ringing anyone I knew who might want some trainers. Over a two week period I sold them all, making a profit. The neighbours must have thought I was running either a drug den or massage parlour as I had males and females coming to my house from 9.00am in the morning until 10.00pm at night.

I phoned my contact and asked for some more. He told me he would deliver the next load the following week. Two days before the delivery I was getting telephone calls from the people who had bought them from me, complaining that the soles were falling off and the stitching was coming apart. There was no way that I was going to repay the money as I had spent it on food and paying bills.

I spoke to the bastard who passed them on to me and he said, 'Paddy, I have just found out they are all fakes shipped in from China.'

I wondered why they had been so cheap. I had

to come clean with all the individuals I'd sold them to, pointing out that was the risk you take when you don't buy from a shop. I then told them I could not refund the money as the contact who supplied them had disappeared.

I used to teach advanced circuit training classes at a local Council leisure gym in the South of Birmingham. I thought I had a great idea. If I bought cheap fitness socks from a warehouse I could re-package them and put them in branded packs. I purchased two hundred pairs of cheap imported Chinese socks for ten pence each. Once I put them in the branded packaging they looked expensive. On the evening of the fitness class I told all the students that the sports socks I was selling were of the highest quality and I was selling them for £2.00 a pack. To my surprise I sold nearly every pair, making a profit of around £1.80p.

The following week, the students approached me complaining that holes were appearing in the heels and toes. I told them that it was probably their trainers, or else they did not cut their toe nails. They believed me, thinking I could well be right. I managed to get away with that one by the skin of my teeth.

One of the students at my boxing martial arts club approached me one evening after a training session and asked me if I would like to make some extra cash. Obviously I asked what it involved. He told me that he could get quality alcohol at one fifth of the price. I jumped at it and asked how many bottles he could get me. I could have as many as I wanted, so I ordered twenty boxes of spirits and sold them for half the price the general public would pay for them in the shops.

Everyone I knew was buying it from me.

After about three months of selling the liquor, I got a telephone call.

'Paddy, that alcohol you're selling is watered down and fake.'

But the funny thing about it was that all my customers were getting pissed on it. Isn't it surprising what a label can do for a bottle?

The funniest one of all was when an acquaintance, Darren, approached me and asked me to call at a house with him to collect some money from a former business partner. I owed Darren a favour so I went along with him to an address in Harborne in the West Midlands. I suggested that Darren stayed out of sight, which he did. We found the address and I hammered on the door. A man in his early thirties opened the door and I immediately grabbed him around the neck and started to threaten him.

'I don't know what you're talking about,' he insisted. I then heard a loud and horrified shout from behind me.

'Paddy, it's the wrong man!'

I apologised to the innocent man and hurried away. I could hear the man shouting out, 'I am calling the police!'

Thank God it was a dark winter's night. When I caught up with Darren I started to give him a bollocking and told him to get his facts right. Then we just pissed ourselves with laughter.

I recently bought a car from a well known dealer. The car was a Volvo V40. When I took the car for a test drive, I did not notice that it had clocked up 60,000 miles. However, when I rang the car trader the next morning, he told me over the phone that there were 50,000 miles on the clock. I thought nothing of it and I went round to his house the next day and agreed on a price. I paid for the vehicle, minus a balance of £450.

As I drove the car home, I then noticed that it had driven 60,000 miles. I rang him on the Sunday morning and told him of his error. He apologised and said he would refund my money. I refused and said that we had to re negotiate the deal. I arranged for us to meet at my gym. He brought the money that I had paid him and said he would like the car back. I refused and said no way.

Due to his error, he knocked off another £100 for me. I know he was not happy about that, but we all know that some car dealers are well known for ripping buyers off. I am sure he has had more good days of earning extra money from his customers than bad days. The vehicle I purchased was an excellent deal. I was just being cheeky to see if I could get the car cheaper, which I did. My point to all this is, stick to your guns as you never know what you might get out of a situation.

I am sure he still made plenty from the deal but not as much as he wanted… and having a meeting in a boxing martial arts club helped.

WUMA WARLORDS KUMITE CHALLENGE RECORD TITLE

The telephone rang. Richard Hopkins, President of the World United Martial Arts Association, was on the other end.

'Hello, Paddy. Fancy breaking the WUMA Warlords Karate Boxing Challenge again that you set way back in 2000?'

I paused for a moment, recalling how much pain I had been through last time. I replied yes, I would have a go. I turned up two weeks later at the Sports Centre in Cheltenham, feeling nervous and wondering if my punch resistance and fitness was up to standard.

The mighty Richard Hopkins came over to me at the event. 'Do your best,' he said, 'the other black belts will be going for a hundred rounds anyway.'

The rules were one-minute rounds and one-minute rest breaks.

I paced myself for the first 25 rounds, but after that I started to step it up. There were some excellent full contact fighters who had previous boxing experience and they gave me as good as they got, with heavy body shots and hooks to my head. At that stage your resistance steps in and you can't feel the pain any more.

By round 80 I was starting to feel it mentally. I was getting more sluggish with each round. Some of the fighters were WUMA World and European champions and they were dishing it out. At last it was the final countdown for the 100 rounds. Usually at this stage of the challenge, a lot of the black belts decide to stop as they have reached their personal goal. I have to admit I was also feeling the pace.

Richard Hopkins looked at me. 'Doyle, do you want to go for the World Record? I can only give you a minute to reply.'

If Richard Hopkins had only known what I was thinking. In my mind, I was calling him every evil name on the planet.

'Ten seconds to decide!' shouted the timekeeper.

I drank some water, put my mouth guard back in and growled, 'Yes.'

They made a ring and my opponents were top WUMA black belts, some of whom were World and European champions. I had to beat 131 contact rounds in 5 hours. They were the hardest rounds I had ever fought. I felt each blow, but I knew I had to stand there and give as good as I got. I collapsed in one of the rounds, landing on my backside. That man Hopkins and one of the officials picked me up and threw me back in. I knew at this stage that I would have to be stretchered out, as I could never leave the circle. Finally the last round came. The spectators were shouting and the hairs were standing up on the back of my neck. I gave it my all. Although I had lost all my power, the last ten seconds came…

... then the final bell. I fell to the ground, feeling totally exhausted. After a few minutes my hand was raised by Richard Hopkins as he proclaimed me the new Warlords Champion, achieving 141 rounds in 5 hours. My body was battered and bruised but it was all worth it. The injuries I received were shin splints, whiplash to the neck, bruised skull and bruised ribs. I was concussed for a week and walking around in a daze, but it was worth every ounce of blood sweat and tears. My respect goes to all of the WUMA black belts I fought on that day. They came to fight and not to lie down.

The World United Martial Arts Association delivers the toughest courses and gradings in the UK and Europe. I remember being at one of their courses along with thirty instructors from around the UK. This course consisted of a challenging circuit training session, pad work using boxing and karate skills, and competitive sparring. When we came to the sparring session we had to fight different instructors. One of them was a karate instructor. When I was fighting him he kept kicking me in the groin. I did tell him that I had no groin protector; nevertheless, he kept on kicking me in my groin. I decided that was enough and I connected with a straight left jab to his mouth. He landed flat on his back. I had managed to cut his lip and dislodge some of his teeth. After receiving first aid, he withdrew from the grading.

Master Richard Hopkins, President of the World United Martial Arts Association UK, said on 24

January 2007:

'I feel that Paddy Doyle does not class himself as an athlete, but as a warrior in life. Everything Paddy decides to go for has to be with the spirit of a warrior and the heart of a bull. Over the years I have seen Mr Doyle go through more pain than one can imagine, just to get him where he wants to be, 'at the top of his field.' He stops for nothing and asks for little. In my eyes, Paddy is what I consider to be a one-off. There is only one Patrick Doyle. The sporting achievements of Paddy Doyle are nothing short of remarkable. The will to win isn't what Paddy is about… I believe it is the strength never to give up that is the essence of Paddy Doyle's success.

'The funniest moment, I feel, over the many years I have known Paddy, was back in 1996 when I conducted an instructor's course at the WUMA HQ in Cheltenham. There were thirty instructors from around the UK. Part of the course involved demanding sparring rounds. During one of the breaks, Paddy whispered to me that one of the karate instructors from Cornwall had been kicking him in the groin, then saying after every foul kick, 'Sorry, but that's what we do at our club.' I whispered back that I believed in doing unto others as they do unto you. Paddy smiled and continued fighting.

'Half an hour later I was called into the hall to administer first aid. Paddy had again partnered the karate instructor and received another three kicks to the groin. Paddy complained and again was told, 'Sorry, but that's what we do at our club.' Paddy decided to heed my words and let fly a left jab into the karate instructor's chin. Down he went and was out like a light, bleeding heavily from the mouth. On waking up, he looked at Paddy and said, 'That was a bit heavy wasn't it?'

Paddy replied, 'Sorry, but that's what we do at our club.'

'Once the instructor had gone home we had a right laugh about it, at his expense, and all the instructors there agreed that he well deserved it, as he also kicked other instructors in the groin when they were fighting. I will never forget that day and always think of it with a smile. I finally want to add that it is an honour to know and train with a student that works so hard with no complaint. While in a lesson, Paddy Doyle would run up and down a mountain ten times if you asked him to. As I have already said, there is only one Paddy Doyle.'

Master Richard Hopkins, 7th Dan, Founder of the World United Martial Arts Association, was inducted into the Martial Arts Hall of Fame 1998.

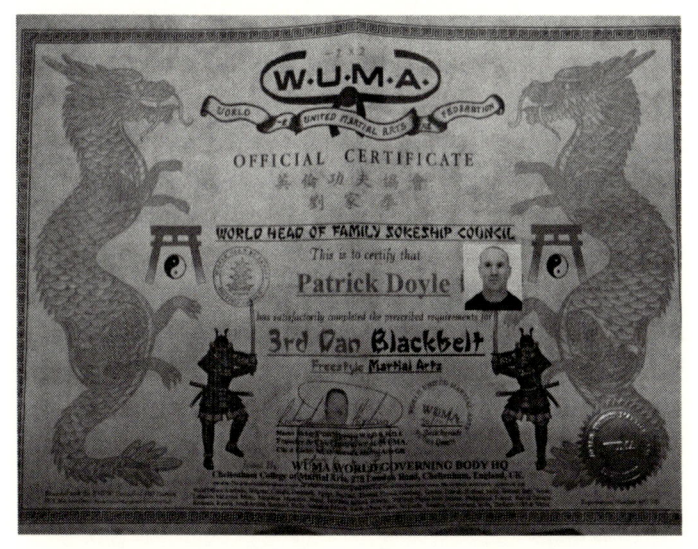

{Official WUMA Black belt 3 rd Dan award}

SPECIAL FORCES SPEED MARCH

I decided to have a crack at the Special Forces Selection Speed March on 26 April 2003. My main pacer was Paul Jones, who is black belt assistant martial arts instructor at my gym. The rest of the support team comprised of Nigel Perry, Brian Perry, Andy and John Norrey, who sadly passed away recently from cancer.

The course involved a 60km speed march over the Brecon Beacons carrying a 55lb backpack. The rules were that I had to be self-supportive and navigate myself over the arduous terrain. I set off with my pacers Paul and Andy at 5am. We speed marched up Pen y Fan which, at 886m/2,907ft, is one the highest mountains in South Wales.

When we got to the top we were hit with low clouds and poor visibility. I then had to navigate the three of us off the steep path. For only a brief second we looked over the side of the path and saw a 200m sheer drop. At this stage I had to make sure my compass bearing was spot on, otherwise we would be knocking on death's door. We had to move quickly as the previous military record was 16 hours, plus the support team were waiting for us at the first checkpoint to verify my time and make sure I was keeping to the route. As the day went on, my legs were burning and I was developing skin sores on my back. The weather was typical; one minute it was calm, the next it was strong winds and heavy rain.

At each checkpoint we had a hot drink and swiftly carried on to the next stop off point. Every couple of miles I was checking my stopwatch. The reason for this was to make sure I was on time and not falling behind. As the day wore on we were all tiring. The backpack was now really digging into my shoulders and lower back.

At last, Nigel Perry who was waiting at the last checkpoint said, 'You have only three miles to go.'

As I checked the map, the contours were very close and I remember thinking when will this end? I could see the last checkpoint. I put my head down and dug in and went for the finish line, and when I crossed it and sat down, the steam was coming off my body. The official time was called out by John Norrey; it was 14 hours 50 minutes. I climbed into the support vehicle and collapsed. We made our way back to the hostel and had a shower. Nigel, who was a chef in a former life, cooked us a curry. We were all desperately hungry, although the curry tasted like diesel and the rice resembled plaster.

We gulped it down, not worrying about the consequences, but thank God Nigel gave up his career as a chef… he did humanity a favour. My joints and muscles were aching for about a week afterwards. I sustained blisters on both feet, skin sores on my back and a torn calf muscle.

Graham Petrie, Ex Reserves Army Regiment Corporal Instructor. `I first met Doyle in 1981 as a 17 yr old recruit training for recruit selection for a specialised Reserves Unit. I was a Corporal Instructor. Doyle stood out initially for two reasons, number one being what appeared to be a home made tattoo on his arm and secondly his eyes, which were darting in all directions, busy weighing up opportunities and possibilites. In the arduous training that followed he was again outstanding for the right reasons, perseverance, fitness but most of all his sheer determination and refusal to quit.

This was exemplified by the boots issue, when he limped into a checkpoint on Brecon Beacons late at night. I enquired in a ` caring` manner about his problems as he had one boot on and the other boot off. His standard issue boots were too small and he did not know whether it hurt more to walk with his boots on or without them, hence the removal of one boot. Paddy still completed the training in spite of this difficulty where lesser men would have quit.

Due to Paddy Doyle's outstanding natural fitness, determination, aggression and will to win we recommended he join the regular Parachute Regiment which he did with great success, winning the trophy for Champion recruit, a natural Para.`

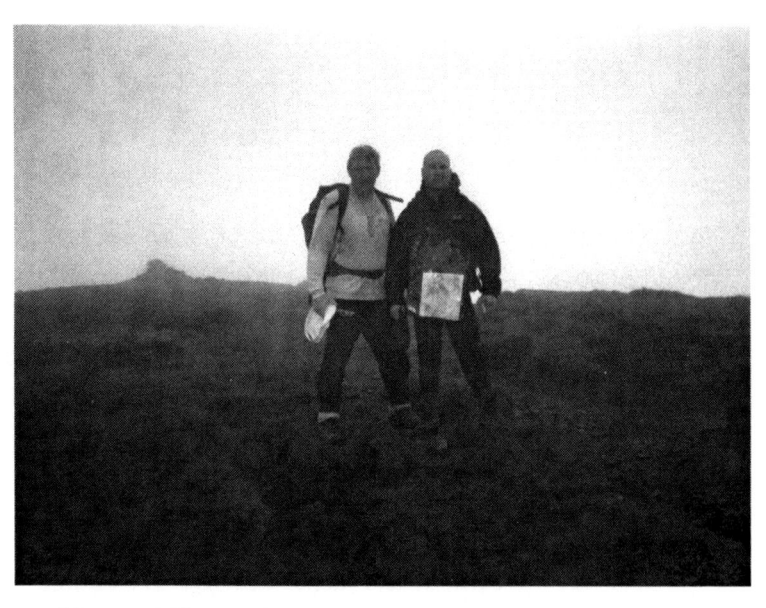

{Special Forces Speed March Record carrying 55 lb back pack, Brecon Beacon Wales, 14 hrs 50 mins}

GUINNESS WORLD RECORDS FESTIVAL, FLENSBURG, GERMANY

I was invited by the German promoters to attempt two fitness endurance records at the Guinness World Records Challenge festival on 13 August 2005. My team members on this occasion were David Chubb and Wayne Ferguson. We were met at the airport and driven for two hours to our destination. When we arrived at the hostel all we wanted to do was rest. The rooms looked like East German prison cells. They were clean but dull and plain.

All I could hear was David Chubb's voice. 'What the hell is this? I've come all the way from Birmingham and been asked to sleep in a prison cell?'

Wayne was laughing and so was I. But I had to concentrate on the World Records and forget about the rooms.

The next day I met up with the promoters and organisers and was told what time I would be attempting the World Records. The first challenge was the most martial arts punches in one minute. The record for this stood at 347, held by Anthony Kelly (Australia.) Wayne Ferguson volunteered to hold the punch pads for me.

The Guinness World Record officials gave me the countdown and I started to punch as fast as possible.

The support was tremendous. The timekeeper shouted stop, and the total was read out over the microphone, 'The new World Record is 470!'

I knew I could not celebrate as I had to attempt another fitness record in ten minutes' time. The attempt was the one hour speed fitness record, for which I had to complete six physical fitness challenges of ten minutes duration each, without any rest breaks. The record was assessed on the number of repetitions and distances achieved for each exercise. The fitness disciplines were rowing, cycle, running machine carrying a 40lb back pack, versa climber machine, weightlifting and boxing punches (hitting punch pads.)

I started to feel it on the last exercise. The sun was blazing down on my head and cramp started to affect both my calves. Big Dave Chubb was shouting down my ear. 'Come on, Paddy!' he urged, 'Dig in, you are nearly there.'

At last the Guinness official shouted time. I just collapsed on the ground, and after a few minutes got up onto my feet. I was then called up to the stage area where the results were announced to the German spectators and the official awarded me two Guinness World Record certificates. I made a short speech thanking everyone, including my helpers. I then made my way back to the newly-named hostel, which we now called the Prison Cells. The three of us got cleaned up and went out to celebrate in a quiet local bar. We had a steak dinner and some bottles of red wine.

We then made our way to one of the popular bars

where we drank all evening. I could feel the German lager getting into my system. Bursting for a piss, I decided to go to the Gents. When I was in the toilet, a big German geezer stood next to me and started pushing me out of the way, telling me to move myself. I went back a few steps, pissing on the floor. I could not believe what he had done as I was minding my own business. He probably thought that as I was smaller than him, he could bully me. I asked him why he had pushed me so aggressively out of the way and his answer was 'Fuck off.' At this stage, my patience ran out, so I decided to punch him right on the nose.

When I connected, his nose poured with blood and he fell into the corner, holding his nose. I helped him up off the floor to hit him again. I punched him and he accidentally landed onto the floor again. Then two of his friends walked into the toilet and saw him on the floor. I explained what happened. 'If you want some as well, let's go for it,' I said. I was wasting my breath as they could not speak English. They were sizing me up when David Chubb came in and saw what was going on.

The German who was crouched in the corner was bleeding heavily. His blood adorned the ceiling as well as the floor. David said, 'Come on, Paddy, let's get the fuck out of here.'

We legged it out of the bar, back to the hostel. Talking about it later, we realized that if we had stayed in the bar, they could have rung some of their friends and possibly have been waiting for us outside with baseball bats. The next morning we were dropped off at the airport. I was thinking what if it had been reported to the Police? They would have my description, but luckily enough that did not happen and we landed back at Birmingham Airport safely and still in one piece.

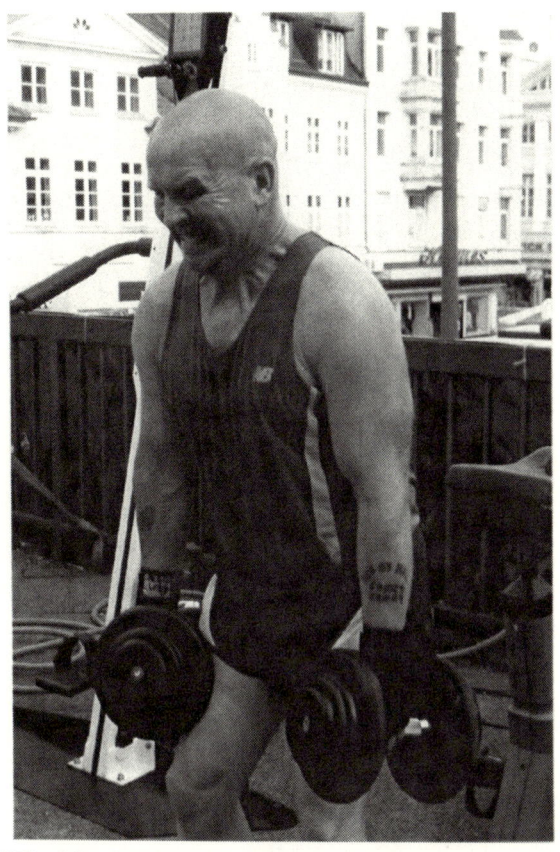

{ World 1 Hour strength speed fitness record, 6 ten minute challenges. Flensburg Germany. 13th August 2005}

WORLD FITNESS CHAMPIONS RECORD TITLE 27ᴴ FEBRUARY 2006

I decided that this was going to be my last ultra fitness record challenge, and I would stick to shorter distance World Fitness Records in future. World Record Titles of this magnitude mentally and physically wreck you, and the injuries last a lot longer. An American athlete, whom I had already beaten, held the previous World best time which stood at 18 hours 15 minutes 2 seconds. The physical fitness challenges I had to complete in the fastest time were:

- 2-mile and 21 metre swim
- 20-mile row
- 10¼-mile run
- 20¼-mile cross trainer
- 10-mile speed march (25lb back pack)
- 100¾-mile cycle
- 550 star jumps
- 3010 sit-up crunches
- 505 hanging leg lifts
- 300,000lb weightlifting (various upper body lifts only)

I was paced and supported by Military Access students from Solihull College UK. They were a great support and were pushing me all the way. I remember feeling tired at the halfway point. My joints were stiffening up and I started to close my eyes. But years of pushing my body and my strength of mind got me through it. The last three hours of the record were crucial. I had to stay focused. The crowd started to build up and the shouting was getting louder. This helped me to push my body to the maximum.

When I was on the rowing machine, Nigel Perry and Paul Jones were passing me water and telling me to stay sharp. I had a quick water break and acknowledged David Chubb and his girlfriend, Kerry, in the crowd. The one thing I must not do now was stop or slow down. I had 10,000 metres left on the rower and I gave it my best. What looked like sweat pouring down my face was in fact a deluge of tears. No one knew the pain I was going through.

My mind was pushed to the limits; everything seemed to be a bleary vision. Finally, one of the officials shouted, 'Paddy, you only have 1,000 metres to go!'

It was the longest 1,000 metres ever. I finally reached the 20-mile target and collapsed onto the floor. The spectators were still shouting at the top of their voices. The MC read out the official time, 'Ladies and gentleman, the new World Record is now 17 hours 12 minutes and 33 seconds.'

I had beaten the previous World best time by over an hour. I went round all of the spectators and shook their hands. I was then awarded the official certificate and trophy.

A lot of spectators were waiting for me in the bar area. I bought drinks for some of them and talked about how I felt. My body was in bits for about three weeks afterwards. I was on another planet. As I have said before, World Titles of that level affect your mind and body. All I wanted to do was sleep.

GLEASON'S BOXING GYM BROOKLYN NEW YORK 5 AUGUST 2006

Although I have achieved some tough, challenging World Fitness Endurance Records abroad, this was the most nerve racking. I felt that the USA was *the* place to prove myself in the world of physical endurance, and a lot of the Guinness World Records fitness records were held by American athletes. I was nervous throughout my training… what if I suffered an injury?

A good friend of mine, Joe Egan, who is a former professional boxer and number one sparring partner to Mike Tyson, advised me to contact Bruce Silverglade, the owner and boxing promoter of Gleason's. I emailed Bruce three months in advance to ask him if I could use Gleason's for my Debut World Ultra Fitness Record. He agreed straight away. The main official who then helped me to set it up was the Great Throwdini, who is the holder of seven knife-throwing World Records, one USA National knife-throwing title and the former holder of two World Championship titles. His real name is Doctor David Adamovich, and he was the main lynch pin in organising the accommodation and the documentation to authenticate the World Record on completion.

I arrived in New York and David picked me up from the airport. He drove me to his home where I met his wife Barbara and their beautiful dog, Phantom. We got down to business and started to plan for the big day. David already had my diet sorted out and told me he had arranged for fellow American sports-qualified judges to adjudicate the event.

Finally the morning came. I was up at 6am getting my kit ready and planning in my head how I would approach the challenge. My reason for this was because 5th August happened to be falling on a heat wave and Gleason's did not have an air- conditioning system, only a standard fan. I knew I would have to dig deep mentally to block out the extreme heat.

I arrived at Gleason's feeling uptight but ready to go. Bruce Silverglade showed David and me round the gym, and then I started to prepare myself mentally for the record. The American support team arrived.

The countdown came... 5... 4... 3... 2...1 and I was off. The first physical fitness challenge was running on the treadmill carrying a 40lb backpack. I paced myself for the first ten minutes before stepping up the pace, and finishing with a total distance of 5½ miles. I was allowed a 3-minute rest break and then started the shuttle sprints, carrying the same weight. The distance was 30ft, but at this stage the lack of air conditioning was starting to affect me. However, the American support team were brilliant. Ben Lerer, Mike Rothman and Harry Munroe were constantly shouting encouragement, which helped me tremendously. It motivated me to block out the heat. At last I finished the full hour, completing 512 sprints. The officials allowed me another 3-minute rest break, during which I shoved down my throat plenty of strawberries and bananas, which eased the cramp in my calves and quads. The standing chest press was next. I had to push out a 30lb dumbbell for another hour. My elbows were feeling it when I locked out the weight. The sweat was dripping down my legs and, where I was standing, it looked as though someone had poured two pints of water over me.

At last the official shouted time and I went for a quick piss, escorted of course by an official, and then started the step-ups carrying a 40lb back pack. My legs at this stage were like lead. The salt from the sweat was getting into my eyes and I had to make sure I did not miss a step on the bench, otherwise I would have landed flat on my face or damaged my knees. I knew I had one more fitness exercise after this, so I did not care if my legs seized up as I would have enjoyed it. I suppose that is where my mind kicks in; when the pain gets too much I can block it out and think of the consequences afterwards.

The official again shouted, 'Time!' Another 3-minute break and I started the gym cycle. The boxers and one of the trainers at Gleason's started to gather around and motivate me for the last twenty minutes of the cycle. The last few seconds ticked away and then it was all over. I thanked all the USA World Record team for their help throughout the World Record, and I was then awarded an official World Record Certificate by Doctor David Adamovich and Bruce Silverglade.

When I got back to David's house I had a shower, and some champagne, or a beer. I had a sleep for a couple of hours and then started to reflect on how the day had gone. That same evening David introduced me to his famous aunt, Tanya Adamovich. She qualified for the United States Olympic Team in 1972 and fenced in Munich. In 1973 she then won the United States National Championships. Tanya was also a member of the US World Championship Team competing against Olympic Champions from Europe and Worldwide. It was an honour to meet such an athlete and a kind lady. She told me about her experiences throughout her competitive career and the people she had met. Needless to say, I could have listened to her all day. She was an inspiration.

Dr David Adamovich, in 2007, had these kind words to say:

'As a World Record Holder myself, I first found out about Paddy as being one of the most prolific record holders for all of the World Record Bodies. I was stunned and amazed to find out that one man could achieve so many physical fitness records, by both setting and beating other World Record holders at their own game. Mentally, I envisaged a well-muscled moulded or chiselled boxer versus that of a heavy weight champion or weightlifter who exhibits build and definition. To my surprise, he was neither. In fact, he appears rather normal in body build; fit, but no different from most people working out in a gym.

'What makes Paddy different is his genetic and muscle fibre make up. He is different from the normal person. He feels the pain of intense lactic acid build up as his muscles are pushed far beyond the imaginable.

But his ability to withstand that pain and work through it is what makes him stand out. Everyone else feels the pain, decides it's too much and yields. Paddy feels the pain setting in, and sets his goals on the other side. He has an uncanny ability to focus past the finish line. The average person sees pain and resets the goal to the immediate. Paddy sees the pain and resets the goal to the future.

'One remarkable thing I recall is that when he finished the fifth hour of his World Endurance Record at Gleason's, his face was full of pleasure. He passed the finishing line and immediately turned to everyone there and began congratulating them for helping him. No Pain no glory? Yes, that's his motto but he doesn't show the pain. He just takes the glory. I had tears in my eyes with fulfilment of the moment and the World Record. I did my best to hide them but could only do so as I congratulated him with a loud round of applause'.

OFFICIAL WORLD RECORD CERTIFICATE

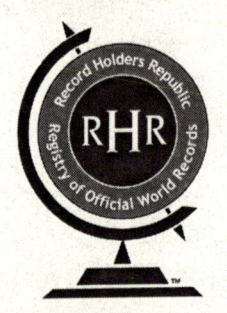

www.recordholdersrepublic.co.uk

WORLD ULTRA FITNESS CHALLENGE

On August 5, 2006, **PADDY DOYLE** of Balsall Common, UK, set the 'World Ultra Fitness Challenge' at Gleason's Gym, Brooklyn, NY, by performing the following 5 one-hour events with a 3 minute break between events:

Treadmill run with 40 lb. back pack: 5.05 miles

Shuttle Run: 30 feet with 40 lb. back pack: 2.91 miles

Standing Chest Press: 30 lbs.: 713 repetitions (716-3)

Steps Ups: 12 inch with 40 lb. back pack: 835 steps

Cycle Ergometer: 0 resistance: 21.6 miles

Mr. Doyle's starting weight was 181.5 lbs. His ending weight was 178.5 lbs. He consumed 6.53 lbs of liquid and 3.0 lbs. of fruit. His net body weight loss was 12.53 lbs. (3 + 9.53). The outside temperature measured 100° Farenheight. The gym was not air-conditioned and used exhaust fans only. Start time 9 AM, finish time 2:12 PM. This astonishing event marks Mr. Doyle's 140th regional, national or world record.

{World 5 hour Ultra Fitness Record Gleasons Boxing Gym, New York}

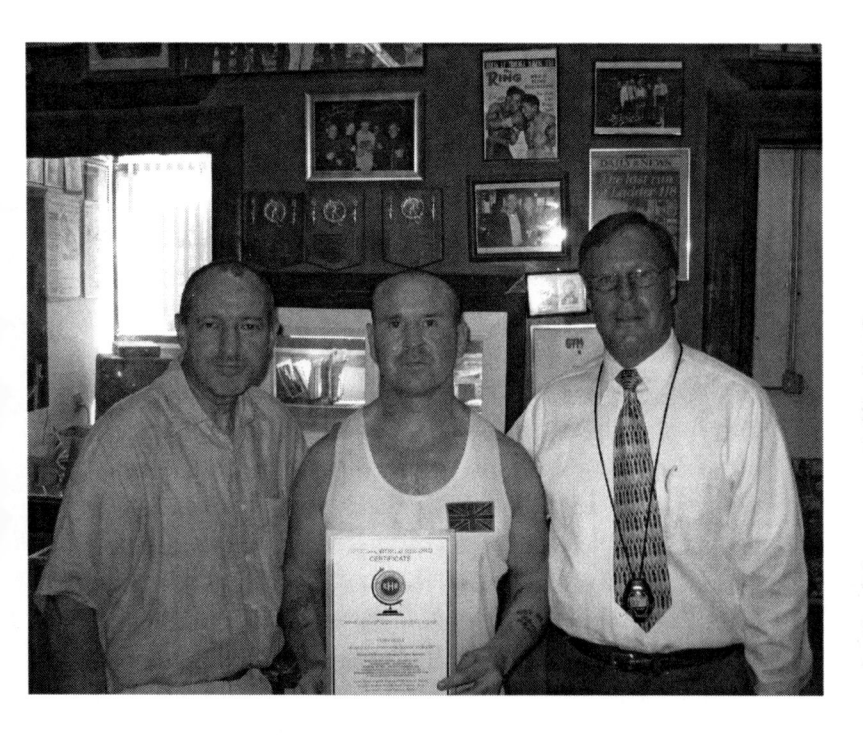

{Left to right Bruce Silverglade, owner of Gleasons Boxing, Paddy Doyle and Dr David Adamovich RHR World Record President}

STRENGTH STEP-UPS CARRYING 56LB BACK PACK

I recovered very quickly after New York and was itching to get back into training. I spoke to my support training team and they suggested that I attempt the step-ups challenge, carrying a 56lb back pack on a 15-inch high bench. My training consisted of speed marching carrying a 90lb back pack, intense boxing sparring, circuit training and doing the step-ups with the same weight. The local BBC Coventry and Warwickshire radio station contacted me and invited me to attempt the World Record live at their studios. This was great news. The date was set and the new World Record was to be attempted on 9 November 2006. I arrived with my support team feeling very, very nervous. You would think after twenty years of achieving numerous strength, speed and stamina challenges that I would be calm. I was quite the opposite. I remember walking up and down in the corridor, wearing the carpet out. Desi Clifton, my loyal friend and coach, winked his eye at me and ordered me to stay focused. Another team member, Nigel Perry, was organising the paperwork in the background and, to my surprise, he looked more nervous than I was.

The BBC Officials gave me five minutes to get ready. The back pack was weighed and Paul Jones, my assistant, put it on my back. The first one hundred step-ups were not a problem, but once again the bloody heat got to me as there was no air conditioning. Spectators and supporters started to turn up at the studios and, once again, their shouting helped to spur me on. Big Dave Chubb was in the background, staring straight at me and this helped me to cut out the pain and just give it my all.

The timekeepers called out five more minutes to go. I was determined not to stop, for the crowd just kept cheering and urging me on to the finish. Then one of the timekeepers shouted time, and the BBC radio presenter Bob Brolly shoved a microphone into my face and asked me how I felt. It took a few seconds to get my composure back. My reply was that at the twentieth minute my back and legs had felt like iron bars, but all my preparation for the attempt had paid off. My girlfriend Deborah came over and kissed me, giving me a big hug.

We then went back to my house with some of the support team and had a few bottles of wine to celebrate. That same evening I started to feel the after-effects. My knees and lower back were in pain. I felt it especially when I was walking down the stairs and getting sharp pains across the front of my knees. I phoned my Sports Therapist, Deborah Ganderton. She attended to my injuries the next day, advising me to rest and take it easy for a few weeks, which I did.

SITREP

SUMMER 2006

DOYLE STILL NUMBER ONE

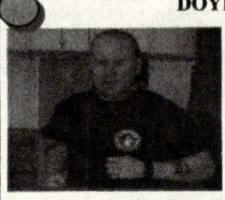

Former Paratrooper Paddy Doyle notched up his 139th fitness endurance record on Sunday 2 July. Doyle a former amateur boxer and full contact martial arts champion, now holds the most officially documented fitness records in the World. He regained his sit up strength records off American James Clarke, a former "USA" Seals Specials Forces soldier. Paddy who is a WASF active unit member regained the following records; . Sit ups in 5 minutes with 50 lb weight on chest total 211 . Sit ups in 10 minutes with 50 lb weight on chest total 351 . Sit ups in 15 minutes with 50 lb weight on chest total 501 . Sit ups in 30 minutes with 50 lb weight on chest total 932 Paddy took on the challenge at the last minute and has been in training for his first World Fitness Record at Gleasons Boxing Gym Brooklyn, New York, he hopes to clinch the World 5 hour Ultra Fitness Record on the 5th August. I'm very nervous because I am going out there without my team so I'm really going into the Lions den," he said. I've taken quite a few fitness records off the the Americans so they want to see me in action. The odds are against me but I'm an endurance athlete so I should be able to travel any where. Paddy's website is www.worldsfittestathlete.co.uk

SOLDIERSPORT

SPORT SHORTS

● THE Paddy Doyle record-breaking machine rumbled on as the former para smashed four more strength and fitness records.

The 43-year-old battled with a chest infection to set the new world bests at the Stamina Boxing and Martial Arts Centre, in Birmingham.

Wearing a 40lb backpack and working to a one-hour time limit, Doyle completed 1,619 step-ups before powering through 663 back-of-hand press-ups and 901 shuttle sprints over 30 feet.

Doyle then set a seven-hour world endurance strength record.

His exploits took the fitness guru's total haul of career strength, speed and stamina bests to 168, 74 of which are world records.

SOLDIER - Magazine of the British Army

MAGAZINE OF THE BRITISH ARMY
SOLDIER
FEBRUARY 2008 £2.50

Paddy's power
Super-fit Doyle makes new assault on world bests

FORMER paratrooper Paddy Doyle pushed his endurance record breaking to the limit by setting four new world bests in one day.

Taking part in the Guinness World Records Day, Doyle was cheered on by a 150-strong crowd at Birmingham's Stamina boxing gym as he broke three existing records and set a new one.

He got off to a good start by performing 1,940 back-of-hand push-ups in one hour, smashing Canadian Doug Pruden's previous best of 1,781.

Hungarian Attila Horvarth was next to lose his record after Doyle upped the world best for circuit training squats in 60 minutes to 4,708.

A total of 5,750 full contact roundhouse martial arts kicks gave the ex-Army man his third record of the day, but he still had to find the strength to become the first person to complete the world strength fitness test.

Starting with a ten-mile speed march carrying a 56lb backpack, Doyle then completed a 63-mile cycle, 367 back-of-hand push-ups, 633 squats and 830 full contact roundhouse martial arts kicks in seven hours to claim his fourth and final world record.

Doyle has now broken 152 world records for strength, speed, stamina and martial arts. ■

SOLDIER - Magazine of the British Army

MARTIAL ARTS AND BOXING PUNCHING WORLD RECORDS 19 JANUARY 2007

My injuries cleared up after the step-ups record and I wanted to increase my Physical Fitness records to an all-time high. The reason was that some American athletes were slowly catching me up, and I wanted to keep my World Number One ranking for having the most fitness endurance records under several different sporting categories. My Press officer sent out a press release saying that I was going to attempt twenty fitness endurance records throughout 2007. I trained all over the Christmas holiday, even Christmas and Boxing Day. After the New Year's holiday I contacted the Guinness Book of World Records and they forwarded me the current result for the World Record for the most martial arts strikes in one hour. This was 11,557 contact strikes, held by Anthony Kelly of Australia. I was also informed by the Alternative Book of Records that there was a current World Record for the most boxing upper cuts in one minute held by Jim Hoover of the USA, which was stood at 333. I knew if I trained hard enough, I could beat the two official World Records. I spoke to my training team and the date was set for 19th January.

Tickets were sent out to my supporters and the word spread that I was going to attempt the two records on the same night. The support team were Colin Dickinson, Paul Jones, Nigel Perry, Brian Perry and David Chubb. Finally, 19th January came and I was ready to go for it. The venue was Stamina's Boxing Gym based in Erdington, UK.

All of the team arrived and assembled. They were all briefed and feeling nervous as they had a lot of responsibilities. David Chubb was appointed to hold the punch pads for the two record attempts, the first of which was the boxing upper cuts in one minute. I knew I had only one shot at this record and my mind and body had to be relaxed. Colin Dickinson, the official timekeeper, gave me the countdown, the two counters and David Chubb got into their positions and on the word, GO! I punched as fast as I could. The crowd of spectators were shouting at the top of their voices, which pushed me even further. Suddenly, I was told to stop. I was glad to; my lungs were bursting.

The timekeeper read out the total. 'Ladies and gentlemen, the new World Record is now 586 contact boxing upper cuts, beating the previous World Record by 253.' The spectators roared, cheering me on for the next official World Record. Once again the team got into their positions and the clock started. This was especially tough as I had been given only five minutes to recover from the last challenge. For the first fifteen minutes of the one hour World Record, I remember my arms feeling tired from the boxing upper cuts. I stopped three or four times, and I knew mentally if I continued stopping and having short breaks there was no way I would beat it.

My mind then went up a gear and I just kept punching as fast and as hard as I could. David's whole body was vibrating with every punch; his head and upper body were being pushed back on every contact strike. From the fifteenth minute onwards, I hardly stopped. I was looking down a tunnel, focused on beating the World Record. Dave was motivating me, shouting at me to get angry and dig in. Team assistant Paul Jones shouted down my ear, 'One minute to go.' I punched my heart out, and at last 'STOP!' was shouted.

I collapsed on my knees and the total was read out. Timekeeper Colin Dickinson informed the crowd that the new World Record was 18,372 strikes in one hour, beating the previous best by 6,815 martial arts strikes. I thanked all of my team and the supporters who turned up. Deborah and I made our way home and reflected on how successful it had been. Unfortunately, David Chubb, who had been holding the punch pads, received mild whiplash and suffered headaches for a week from the impact of the punches. My biceps, triceps and all of my back muscles were stiff for seven days. I had a break from training for about ten days, which helped to relax my mind and rest my body.

THE ARDEN CROSS COUNTRY CHALLENGE MARATHON 24 FEBRUARY 2007

This was a gamble, as I had recently achieved two speed records and was attempting another ultra fitness marathon record in a very short space of time. But the pressure was on me. I said earlier on that I had set my sights on breaking twenty endurance records throughout 2007. I spoke to the officials of the Arden Challenge Walk, and they were very keen for me to attempt the 26 mile cross country marathon carrying a 40lb back pack.

For the previous three weeks I had been out most days and evenings speed marching and carrying a 70lb back pack. Previous experience of training with a heavier back pack had shown that it increased my stamina. This was important, especially as it was over challenging, arduous terrain. My support team for this record were students from the Military Access Course based at Solihull College, and my main pacer was my loyal team assistant, Paul Jones.

We all arrived early at the start point. We met the

officials for the first time and were informed about the stop-off points and the weather conditions, which did not look very good. Brian Keates, the Arden Walk secretary, then weighed my back pack which happened to be eight pounds overweight. The excess weight was taken out and we were then ready to start off at 8am. The official checked his watch and set me going.

I started off with my pacers at a brisk pace, but two miles into the cross country marathon we came up against water-logged fields. The water at most stages of the course came up to my knees. This was due to the extra weight I was carrying. My feet were wet three miles into the attempt, which was not a good sign.

My hat goes off to my girlfriend, Deborah, who assisted me and the pacers for the first six miles of the course. We all passed the first check point, assisted by the Arden challenge leader.

I turned to the team escorting me. 'I don't think we will get any more severely water-logged fields or slippery, muddy paths,' I said. I was very much mistaken, for the next five miles were just as bad. I could see it was affecting the Military Access students physically. By the ten-mile second checkpoint, injuries amongst the team had begun to occur and we started to spread out. I carried on with the fresh Arden Challenge leader and left the team behind, thinking that they would catch me up shortly. However, that was a mistake on my behalf as I should have waited for them, but the walking leader insisted we should carry on. We had not much daylight left and the clock was against us.

Sadly, my pacers got lost while they were trying to catch up with me, but I had to carry on regardless. The course was getting worse. Every field, footpath, and hill I walked up was either flooded or thick with wet, foul mud. Every three steps forward I made, I was sliding back six steps.

I reached the third checkpoint and had some refreshments. Now I was assisted by a new walking leader to guide me, and my former Parachute Regiment Recruit Sergeant, Mike Homer, was there to walk in the last nine miles with me. Deborah also decided to do the last nine miles with me. This was such an uplift for me as the previous seventeen miles had been mentally tiring and challenging and at this stage I was also pissed off with losing my main support team.

Fair play to Mike Homer, he kept me talking on the last nine miles. This helped to take my mind off my blisters and the skin sores on my back. I approached the penultimate checkpoint and my loyal friend Barmy Brian Vernum was there with his headbanging brother, Tony. I will not go into the reasons why they have nicknames of that nature. However, they were passing me water which I needed badly, and cheering me on.

Finally, I was told it was the last two miles to the finishing line. I picked up the pace but once again the water and deep muddy paths slowed me down. The last half mile was downhill and we all got to the finishing line within the allocated time. I thanked the officials and Mike Homer for their support. I was then awarded an official diploma from the Secretary which confirmed the new record time of 9 hours and 8 minutes. The officials then decided that if anyone wanted to break it, they must do it in the same month under similar conditions. I would like to attempt it again as I know I could knock at least two hours off that record.

My next worry was trying to find out where the hell the support team was. The officials received a telephone call saying they were back on the cross country course and were making their own way in. I was told afterwards by Paul Jones that they got back to the finishing line in an overall time of 12 hours. The Arden Challenge Walk Committee commented on their website that I had achieved the new course record under very difficult conditions. My body needed a good rest, especially as I had achieved two World Records and one endurance marathon course record in the space of five weeks. My joints were in bits and I felt run down. I rested for two weeks doing nothing.

Four months later, I decided to have another crack at breaking the course record. I knew if I could get a fast start I could beat my last course record time. The officials weighed my back pack. At 6.30am I was given the count down and we were off. The reason for starting a lot earlier was because of the heat. It was forecast that it would get a lot warmer throughout the day. It was important that I got as many miles under my belt as possible for the first three hours.

All was going well until I slipped and bruised my ankle at the twelve-mile stage. Up until then I was on target to beat the previous record time. I knew I had to dig deep once again to push myself for the next twelve miles. I reached the fifteen mile checkpoint in pain and tired. The official pacer informed me that I was on time, adding that if I kept to the same speed I would break the course time.

The heat was starting to get to me, especially at the

twenty-first mile. The back pack was digging into my shoulders and I was drinking a lot of water… although more went over my head than I drank at that stage. I started picking up the pace on the last four miles, escorted by four pacers and various officials. Finally, I reached the finishing line totally exhausted. The official finishing time was 7 hrs, 37 mins, 2 secs. All of the team who helped me came back to my house and had a few beers. After they left, Deborah helped me to put antiseptic cream on my back and shoulders from where the backpack had rubbed into my skin. Some of the blisters were the size of fifty pence pieces, oozing pus and dead skin.

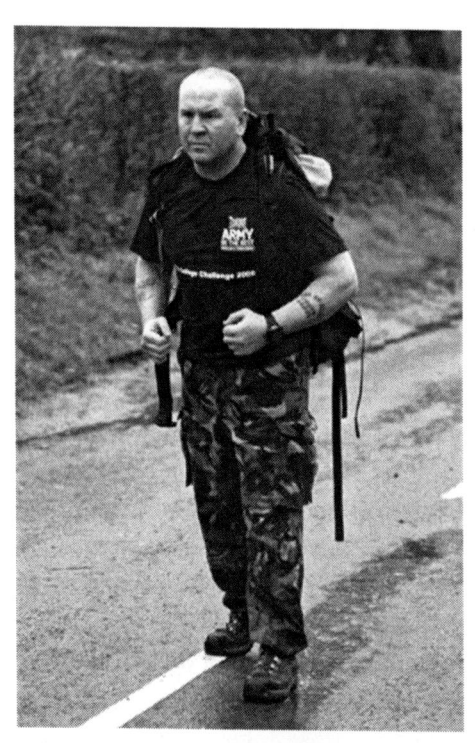

{Arden Challenge Walk Route}

WORLD RECORD BREAKERS CUP CHALLENGE
18 APRIL - 2 MAY 2007

I was once again asked to represent Great Britain in the very first World Record Breakers Cup Challenge, which involved various countries around the World attempting National and World Records. Each country would select a team of athletes and other skilful record holders to amass the most points to win the World Record Cup over a two week period. It was assessed on a points system which is 1 point for setting a record, 2 points for breaking an existing personal record, and 5 points for breaking the opposition's record. There were organised events around the UK throughout the 2 weeks, attempting numerous records. However, I decided to go to the USA and attempt my official records alongside the USA team, hoping to meet my new arch rival, James Clarke, who took six records off me. I arrived at New York's JFK airport on 17th April. World Record senior judge, David Adamovich, picked me up from the airport and drove me back to his place, where I stayed for the next five days.

I knew I had to have an early night as I was naturally

feeling jet-lagged, plus I was informed that I would be attempting some of the World Records the next day at the Record Holders' HQ, New York. The pressure was on and I wanted to give one hundred percent for my country. The 18th April came and I felt very nervous. My game plan was to go for as many speed records as possible. If I went for endurance records, which consisted of going for long periods of time, the points for Great Britain would have been low. In addition I would have picked up injuries at an earlier stage. I found out that the World Record for the most records in one hour was three, currently held by Ashrita Furman (USA.) I had trained very hard for this challenge in the UK and I was aiming to break fourteen records within the hour. The first eight records were speed strike martial arts punch records held by martial arts instructors in the USA. I successfully beat them and then went on to set six fitness speed medicine ball records. The weight of the ball was 10lb.

The points were added up by the adjudicator and totalled 51 points, putting Great Britain at the top of the table. I felt mentally and physically tired after the intensive hour, but I still had to stay focused for the one-hour step-ups record which I was going to attempt in two days' time, at the famous Coney Island Sideshow Theatre in Brooklyn. This venue was the main event for the USA Record holders to break records and increase their points.

Over five records were broken and one USA record holder failed his football attempt. Finally, my name was called and I was introduced to the spectators. To my surprise, I got a rousing cheer. David Adamovich informed the crowd of what I was going to attempt.

The previous World Record which I set on 9 November 2006 was 716 step-ups carrying a back pack. If I were successful in breaking this record I would have gained two more points for Great Britain.

To be honest I was nervous and lonely, as I was used to having my own team around me. I knew no one at the Coney Island Exhibition centre. I was only aware of the spectators and the appointed counters who were assisting me throughout the attempt. My mind kicked in and I just had to adapt and dig deep, blocking out my surroundings. I was directed into my position and the back pack weighing 40lb was then placed onto my back. The officials gave me a count down of five seconds and I started. The first twenty minutes went well, but going into the twenty-fifth, my legs started to burn. The spectators were shouting non-stop, encouraging me all the way. Eric Sears, the appointed USA World Record counter, was passing me water and a towel to rub me down. Another USA official, Thomas Blacke, informed the crowd of how many step-ups I had achieved at the forty-fifth minute.

'The total so far is 730 step-ups!'

The crowd were cheering even louder as they knew I had broken the World Record. Although I felt mentally and physically tired, I wanted to increase the total of step-ups, putting the record out of reach.

At last the final countdown came. Senior official, Mr Blacke, was encouraging the spectators to get behind me, which they did. For the last two minutes I went as fast as I could, finishing with a total of 911, beating the previous record by 195. It was a relief taking the back pack off; my legs felt like jelly. I thanked all the officials and shook hands with the spectators. I was then awarded two official certificates detailing what I had achieved. I was the only World Record Holder to achieve the most fitness endurance records throughout the Record Breakers Challenge. My final points total was 53 points, ranking me the World's number one in the competition. That event certainly pushed my mind to the limits as I had to stay focused for the whole trip, plus I wanted my country to be first.

As soon as I reached the changing room I collapsed onto the chair. After about ten minutes I went for a cold all-over body wash from a sink in the unisex toilet. I stripped off, filled up a bucket of cold water and poured it all over myself. I repeated that four or five times, since it was only the way to clean myself and get rid of the sweat, as there were no showers. As I was busily pouring buckets of water over myself, a queue was forming outside the toilet. As this was the only unisex toilet in the building, men and women were waiting to do their Number Ones and Number Twos, and some were probably desperate.

So they were hammering at the door not realising that I was stripped naked and pouring cold water all over me. They became angry, 'What the fuck are you doing, man?' I knew I had to hurry up but, tired and mentally wrecked after breaking sixteen fitness endurance records in the space of two days, I selfishly replied, 'Oh just fuck off!' Finally, I opened the door and these people with their legs crossed realized who I was; they were the spectators who had been watching the World Record event. They then understand why it took twenty minutes for me to come out. I remember thinking this could only happen in New York.

I informed the officials that I was going for a short walk to find a coffee house. As I was walking round the corner from the venue, a car pulled up and asked me if I wanted some crack/drugs. I replied in a negative way, 'Go fuck yourselves.' It occurred to me that the way I was walking, after achieving one hour of step-ups carrying a 40lb back pack, I probably looked as though I needed some crack. Achieving sixteen endurance and speed records within forty-eight hours was taking its toll. I was still very tired after the long flight over to New York. But I proved to myself and others that a genuine athlete who has a strong mind can travel abroad, adapt and get on with the challenge, regardless of the conditions.

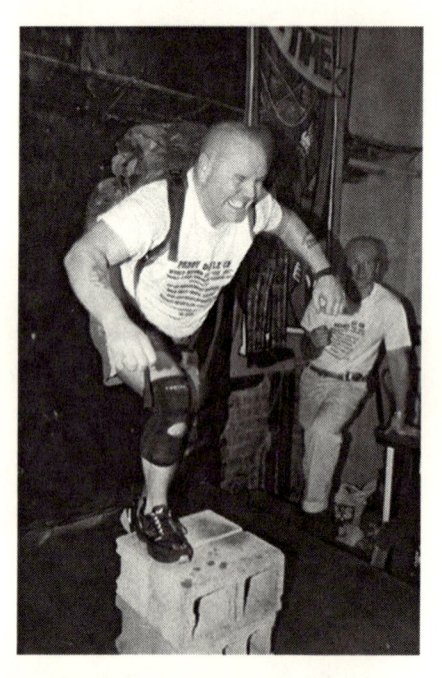

{911 step ups carrying 40 lb back pack in 1 hour, World Record Holders Cup Challenge Coney Island}

GUINNESS WORLD RECORDS DAY 8 NOVEMBER 2007

The pressure was really on to break four demanding endurance fitness records on Guinness World Records Day. My training had gone well in the gym. Paul Jones, who holds a black belt in freestyle martial arts, and my training partners, Matthew Petrie, Ben Goodenough and Carl Brown pushed me to the limits to get myself mentally prepared for the big day. On the build-up to the challenges I was speed marching carrying a 50lb back pack for around three hours, eight to ten rounds of full contact boxing martial arts sparring, strength circuit training workout for one hour, and finishing off with four rounds of bag work.

Three of the Guinness World fitness endurance records were one hour each in duration. The first record was for the most back-of-hands push ups in one hour, held by Doug Pruden (Canada.) I had to beat 1,781. This was especially tiring on the forearm muscles, shoulders and lower back. My team gave me a good motivational talk to get me fired up. This helped me to focus and give it my best. I was suffering at the thirty-minute stage, doubting whether I'd be able to beat it. However, one of the officials shouted out that my total so far was 1,386. That gave me a boost as I knew then that I had beaten Doug Pruden's thirty-minute record and I was well on my way to clinch the Guinness record. The countdown finally came; the judges told me I had one minute to complete the full hour. Time was shouted at last and the result was given out by the Official, 'The new World Record is 1,940 back-of-hands push ups!'

Next up was the dreaded squats record held by Attila Horvarth (Hungary.) The record stood at 4,656 in one hour. I knew this was going to be a challenging record to beat, but I had trained hard for it and was hungry to smash it. At the half way stage my calves and quad muscles were tightening up. My training team kept shouting at me, this helped me to keep my speed constant and block out the pain from my legs, glute muscles and knees. I was pleased that I had worked hard in the gym, concentrating on building up my quad muscles, which paid off.

At last the countdown came. This was one World Record I did not want to attempt again. The official read out the results to the supporters, 'The new World Record is 4,708!' The crowd applauded and I then started to prepare for the next challenge.

The news did not sink in at first as I had to get myself mentally ready for the next World Record, which was for the most full contact kicks in one hour, held by Ron Sarchian (USA) which stood at 5,545 kicks. Although my arms were feeling like lead after completing the back-of-hands push-ups, I had to focus on the next World Record. Big David Chubb was appointed to hold the kicks pads. The rules are that the athlete has to kick the pads above waist height. My method was to alternate each leg when kicking the pads.

As the hour went by my legs were cramping up but the supporters were shouting me on. Finally the official timekeeper shouted, 'One more minute to go!' At that stage my legs were burning but I reached the full hour and collapsed on the boxing ring mats. The final total was read out, 'The new World Record is now 5,750 full contact kicks, beating the previous record by 205 kicks!'

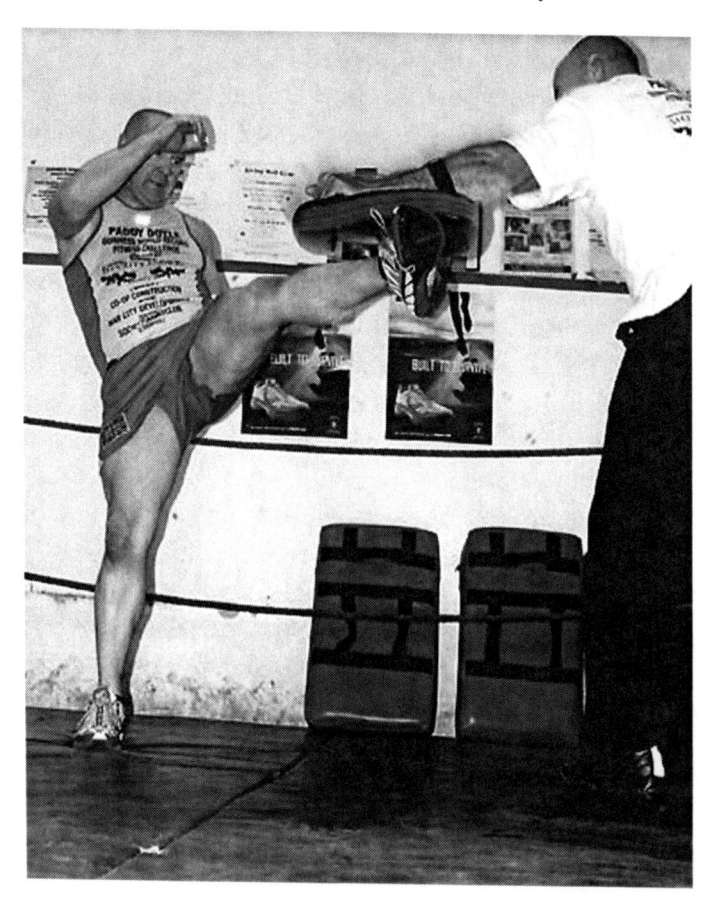

I decided to have a short break and recover from my injuries. I could feel my joints aching and I was mentally tired. This was possibly down to a tough year… I had achieved twenty-four strength endurance speed record challenges. The rest certainly benefited me, as I was ready to go for another official World Record.

I was informed by Guinness World Records that the record I held for the most full contact punches in one hour had been broken. I was totally gutted to hear that. My aim was to get back into the gym and train as hard as I could to take the title back.

The new World Record, which stood at 22,386 full contact punches in one hour, was held by Angelo Breaux (USA). I trained for seven days a week and throughout the Christmas period of 2007. My training went well and my team and I decided to attempt the record on 21 January 2008. I was also aiming to break another record which had stood for twenty years. That record was for the most full contact punches in twelve hours, held by Howard Smith (Wales), which was 121,471 punches.

The day came and my training team and I were ready to go and cut the mustard. The first World Record to attempt was the twelve hour challenge. The appointed officials held the punch pads, the countdown started, and I punched as fast as I could. As each second, minute and hour dragged by, my arms, shoulders and back were cramping up. I knew in my mind that there was no way I would give up. The supporters and officials were encouraging me all the way to the finish.

The timekeeper shouted time and the total of punches was read out. 'The new World Record is now

124,963 punches in a time of 7 hours and 45 minutes!' I was surprised and delighted to have beaten the previous record by 3,492 punches, as well as knocking 4 hrs and 15 minutes off the previous time.

I knew the next main World Record was the one hour challenge. My plan was to dig deep and try not to stop throughout the sixty minutes. The official gave the countdown and I constantly threw punches as fast as I could. Once again, the supporters in the gym were brilliant. They kept shouting, which helped me tremendously. At the twenty-minute stage my arms were feeling weak and tired but my mental strength kicked in, Paul Jones and David Chubb held the punch pads in turn. This kept up my momentum; speed and technique of punching at a fast pace being vital.

Big Dave Chubb shouted two minutes to go. My arms just flew, throwing as many punch strikes as possible. When time was called I collapsed on the floor, breathing heavily. It took some time for the judges to check the final number of punch strikes thrown.

The announcement was read out by Dr Carl Chinn, MBE, who is also Professor of History at Birmingham University and a BBC Radio journalist based in the West Midlands. 'The new World Record is now 29,850 punches in one hour!' I was overjoyed and confess to a few tears in my eyes. Professor Chinn awarded me the trophy and I thanked the supporters for attending. Once checked over by the officials, I travelled home with Deborah and had a bottle of champagne to celebrate my success. My injuries were fairly minor to what I had received in the past. They were only torn biceps. I told myself that I would have a longer break next time to recover from injuries, which did benefit me in the long run.

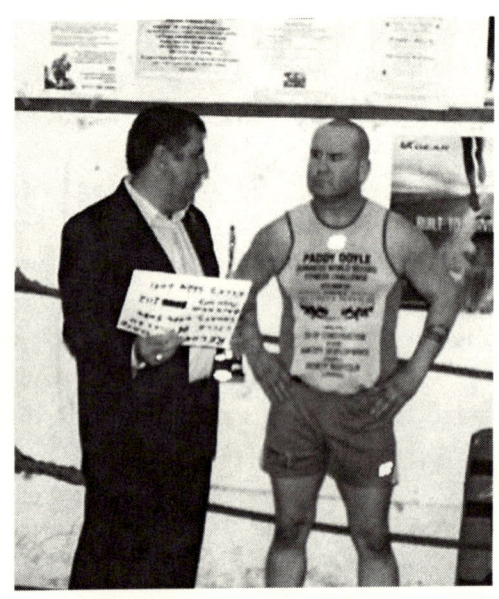

University of Birmingham Professor and Historian Dr Carl Chin Ph.D MBE. Confirming world record Results. Date 8th November 2007}

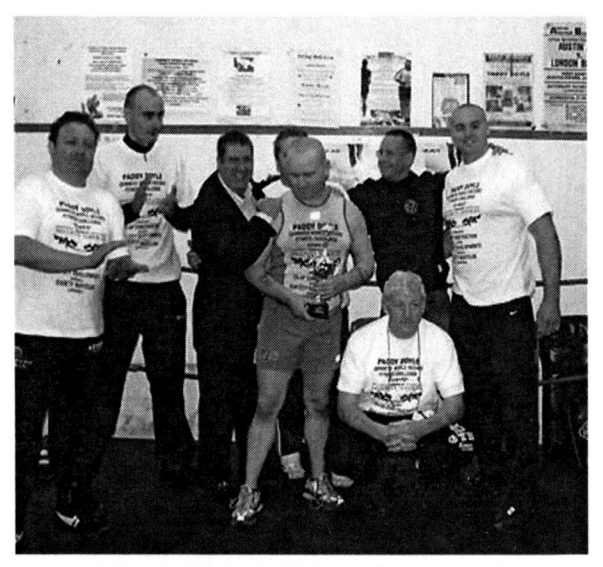

{World Record Team Members}

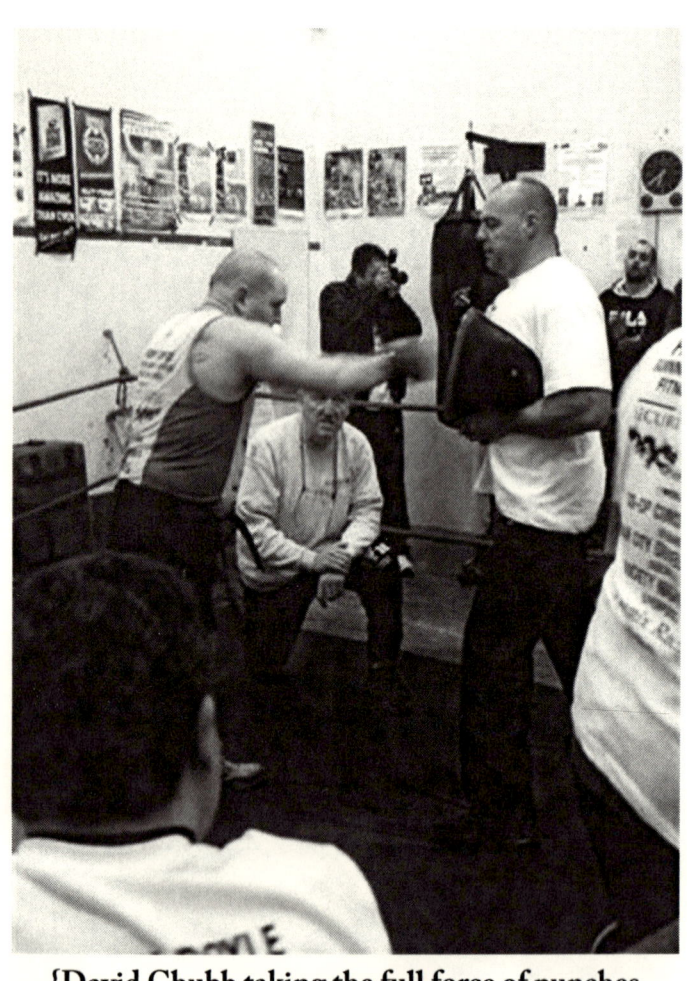

{David Chubb taking the full force of punches thrown in 1 hour by Paddy Doyle. Total 29,850 full contact strikes}

I received a telephone call from the Guinness World Records Head Office in London, asking me if I wanted to attempt a World Record on the Channel 4 Paul O' Grady show. The Guinness World Record was for the most back-of-hands push ups in one minute carrying a 40lb back pack. I was very nervous as I had taken the challenge at short notice, having only three weeks to prepare. I travelled down to London the day before, and the next morning I was driven to the studios. There I met the Guinness officials, who briefed me on the rules and regulations.

I was then escorted onto the stage in front of a live audience. Paul O'Grady introduced himself to me and, along with the Guinness officials, gave me the countdown. Nerves and adrenalin were getting to me. I knew I had to focus and give it my all. At the thirty seconds mark I had a short pain in my lower back, but my mind once again took over and pushed me to the final second. Guinness official, Amarillis Espinoza, read out the total, which was 22 push-ups. I was awarded my Guinness certificate and limped off the stage, trying to conceal my back pain. That injury would come back to haunt me at a later World Record attempt.

After two weeks rest and having had some sports therapy treatment on my back, I was itching to my push my body again and retake another World Record which had been taken from me by a fellow British athlete, Rob Simpson from Leeds (UK). Simpson set an impressive strength step-ups records of 1,511 in one hour on a 15-inch bench carrying a 40lb back pack. I knew I had to train for this record, but my lower back was worrying me. However, my team pushed me on the training nights in the ring, sparring, and also on the circuit training workouts.

We decided to go for two other fitness endurance records on the same day. The date was set: 13 May 2008. The first record to fall was the step-ups record, completing 1,619 in one hour and beating the previous record by 108. I then re – fuelled, got my head focused, and attempted to set a new World Record for the most back-of-hands push-ups in one hour carrying a 40lb back pack. It was the longest hour ever. My arms, back, shoulders and chest were still aching after the step-ups record.

The team around me kept me going and, finally, the last few seconds came and I collapsed on the mat. My final total was 663. My leg muscles were starting to cramp up and my upper body felt weak. My team huddled around me and gave me a pep talk as the next record was for the most 20-metre shuttle sprints in one hour carrying a 40lb back pack. Before I started the sprints I ate a load of bananas, which helped to minimise the cramp in my legs. The pacers were Colin Dickinson and Carl Brown. Throughout the hour I felt like falling flat on my face, but that hunger for success kept me going until the final second. The total of sprints was 901. Afterwards I slept for two days, while my body felt like a concrete block for a whole week. My lower back injury came back to haunt me, since I was having problems bending and walking.

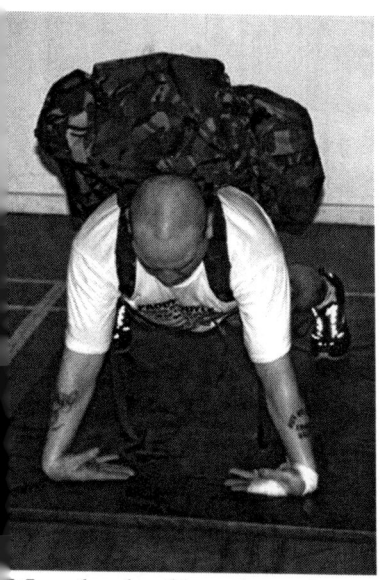

Most back of hands push ups in 1 hour carrying 40 lb back pack - total 663}

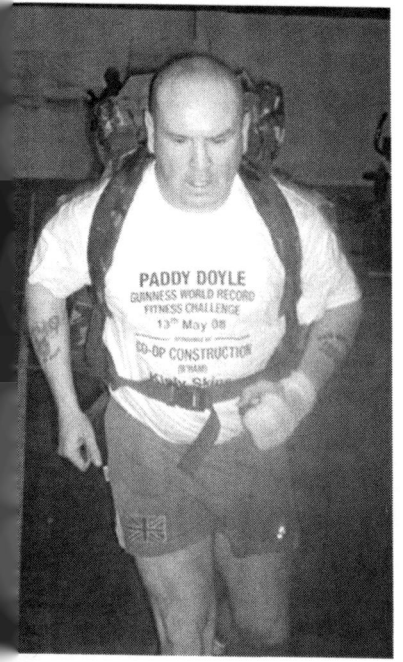

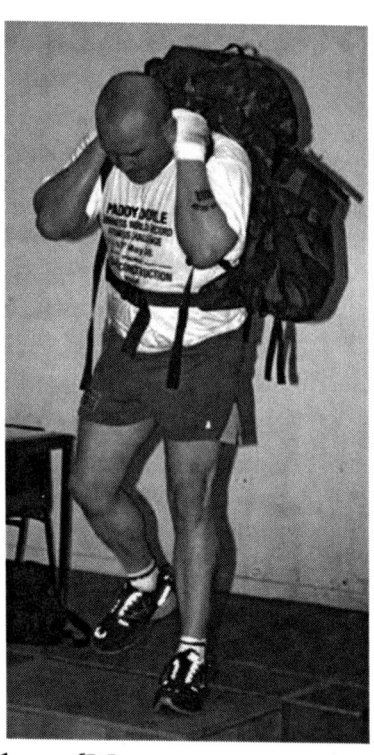

Above: {Most step ups in 1 hour carrying 40 lb back pack on 15 inch bench - total 1,619}

Left: { Most shuttle sprints, distance 30 feet, carrying 40 lb back pack in 1 hour - total 901 sprints}

I was intending to travel to the USA in August to attempt two fitness endurance records, but my back was plaguing me again. Whilst training for the build-up for the record, my lower back finally gave in. I had constant pain down my left leg for some weeks. I went to see John Williams, my osteopath, who said it could possibly be a herniated disc. I thought nothing of it and carried on training, though with some difficulty. I was given the go ahead by Guinness World Records to attempt the one minute back-of-hands push-ups carrying a 40lb back which I had previously set in March 2008.

The World Record was to be held at the Equinox Fitness Club, New York. Danny Girton, the North American Guinness Records official, was in attendance along with Dr David Adamovich from the Registry of World Record Holders, USA. Once again I was briefed on the rules and regulations by the judges. I was going for two fitness endurance records but my back was telling me no. The pain was affecting me mentally. In the end I decided just to go for the one minute record, and attempt the multi-fitness record on another date. The Equinox club members and fitness coaches started to gather around the matted area and watched with interest to see how I would attempt such a World Record, which had never been seen in the USA before.

I was told to get into position, and the clock started. My aim was to beat 22 back-of-hands push-ups but as each second ticked by, my arms started to seize up. However, the crowd support was great. At last the minute was up and Guinness World Records official, Danny Girton, read out the total which was 30 repetitions. I had beaten my previous record by 8.

I stayed a few more days in New York with some friends and got engaged to my girlfriend, Deborah, an event which finished off our visit to New York with a bang. As soon as I arrived home I went to see my doctor, who referred me to the spinal consultant at Solihull Hospital. After completing a series of tests, he confirmed that I had a herniated disc. That meant that while I was training on the build-up for the World Record and also attempting it, I was doing so with a damaged disc. After reflecting on what had happened in New York, I realized that if had I carried on for the one hour strength record after the one minute record, I could possibly have ended up in a wheelchair.

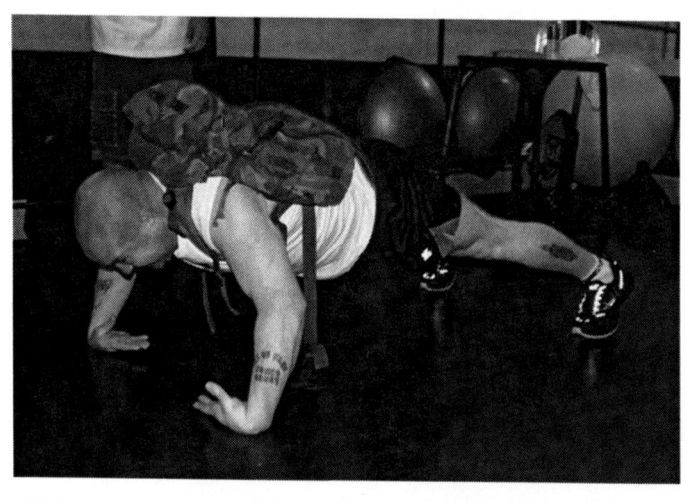

{Most back of hands push ups in 1 minute carrying 40 lb back pack total 30}

MILITARY SPECIAL FORCES TRAINING

There is no doubt that serving in the army helped me to be more focused and disciplined, an experience which has helped me to achieve all of my Fitness Endurance Records and Physical Fitness Challenges. Although I always had that competitive edge, the military definitely put the icing on the cake. I was honoured to be a serving active instructor with the World Association of Special Forces, teaching physical fitness and self defence courses. The Special Forces Association was made up of current serving and former members of the French Foreign Legion, South African, European and British Special Forces soldiers. It was not a mercenary unit, as rumour had it, but an elite military unit/association which trained itself in hostage rescue and close protection.

Many of the men who were members of the Association went on to serve in Iraq, Afghanistan, Congo, and other parts of the world which were suffering from political turmoil. The courses I instructed were attended by some members of the British Army who strongly believed in flying the British flag. Alan Ashes, the senior instructor and founder of the WASF, was a former Paratrooper and Special Forces soldier. He has supported me many times at various World Records. He is a loyal friend and someone you can rely on when the bullets start flying.

I first joined the World Association of Special Forces in September 2000 and the first course I attended was at a Military camp. It was a hostage rescue course and it was very intensive as we had to learn new skills and techniques to storm a building. We were put through various tests such as unarmed combat, assault course and physical fitness. Some members found it very hard when they were doing the fitness exercises, to the extent that they were vomiting as they were running.

After the training, we were split into two teams of four. We then had to plan how to approach the building. We were finally given the go ahead and cautiously made our way into the building, where we had to look for booby traps and check each room for the enemy and hostage. It was a hot summer's day and the gas masks were making it hard for us to breathe or see anything, but we managed to clear each room successfully and extract the hostage. I can remember my knees and elbows bleeding, but that was to be expected.

Six years later, I applied to the Association to become a hostage rescue instructor. The senior course instructor was Roy Mobsby, who was a former Staff Sergeant and Paratrooper serving 35 years in the British Army, and a military adviser to security companies in Iraq and Afghanistan. Roy had a wealth of experience, having completed twelve tours of Iraq, and was wounded on one occasion whilst on operations. He and the Special Forces Instructors certainly put me through it. I was with a good team on the course and I was proud to be awarded the Instructor Certificate at the end of the course.

Alan Ashes, World Association of Special Forces President 2007 had this to say:

'I first met Paddy on a Special Forces Tactics and Rescue Course, run at a former Special Forces military establishment on the south coast of England. The students were made up mainly of ex-UK forces personnel and close protection officers. I remember looking at the personnel on the course with chief instructor and former Paratrooper Roy Mobsby, and remarking jokingly what a motley crew of cut-throats we had on that course.

'As is customary in all military introductions, the first phase is always physical fitness. Two of the students stood out amongst the rest once the course started. One of these students I knew personally from my time in Bosnia. One was an ex-French Legionnaire (he knows who he is,) and the other was Paddy. At that time I had only briefly spoken to Paddy, but his physical fitness had shone through along with his leadership skills in helping fellow students over the assault course. I had noticed for the first time Paddy's wicked sense of humour, especially with one particular student who had a fear of water, which we all thought very strange as this student was an ex-Navy Diver! I got to know Paddy over the next few days of the intensive course, and realised that, as an ex-Paratrooper himself, he had that wicked airborne sense of humour and that determination both in his World Record Fitness Endurance achievements and his military career, to carry on and complete his objectives no matter what the elements and pain barrier threw at him. We have since become very good friends and have met on several of Paddy's World Record achievements. If I had to sum the man up, I would say he is professional, determined and focused but still retains his wicked sense of humour.'

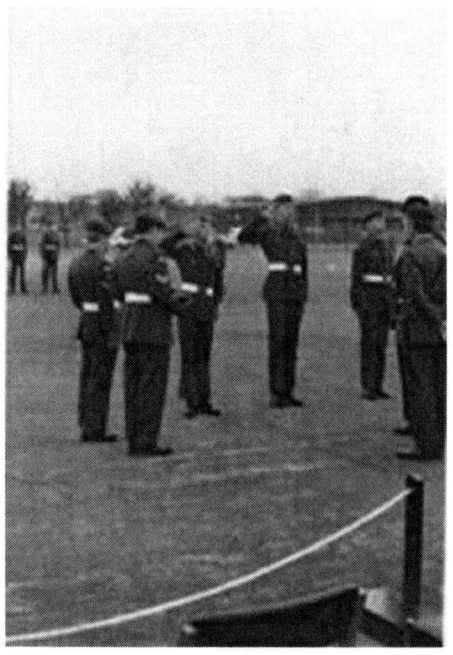

{ Left of Pic, Paddy Doyle being awarded the Champion Recruit of 506 platoon. Parachute Regiment. March 1985}

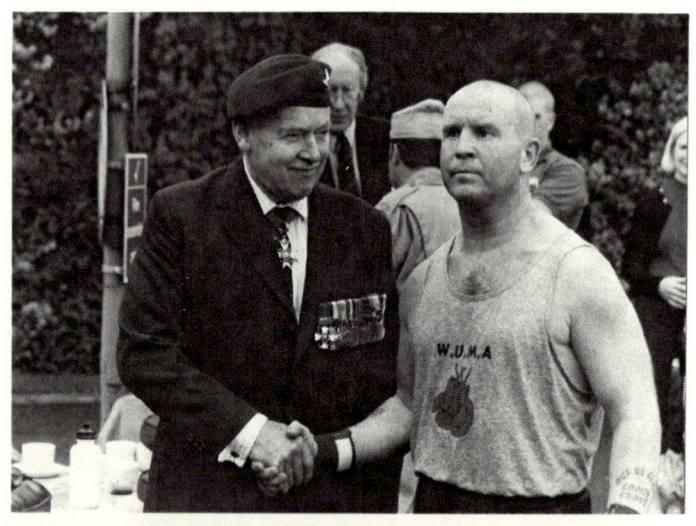

{Congratulated by General Sir Farrar Hockley, achieving the most fullcontact punches , elbow strikes and kicks in 1 hour set on 19 Aug 2001}

TRAINING AND WHAT MAKES ME TICK

I will not go over old ground but, as mentioned in a previous autobiography, I attempt strength speed stamina records purely for the challenge and a personal sense of achievement. Money is a secondary consideration. Many supporters and the media always ask why I do it and how I stay fit and my answer to that is I love pushing my body to the maximum. Running around an athletics track a few times would be boring. When I achieve a fitness endurance challenge I have a week off and get back into training as soon as possible; it is too easy to let yourself go. Consistency is the secret. I always stay on top of my training even if it is only twenty minutes per day. I very rarely run when I am preparing for any physical challenge; I like to go speed marching over cross country carrying a back pack. Sometimes the speed marching can take up to three or four hours, but you can get on with the training and there is just you and the countryside, no roads and no traffic.

Since I have started speed marching on a regular basis, my injuries have reduced. I no longer suffer as I used to from calf and hamstring strains, shin splints and lower back injuries. Power walking has certainly reduced the impact on my joints. I also found out a year ago that certain individuals are born with a stamina gene. This could also be the answer to why I have excellent stamina levels when I am pushing my body, either when I am training or competing to extreme levels. A stamina gene could possibly give me a higher pain threshold than most individuals, helping me to overcome lactic acid build up in my body. I have trained with many well-established and recognised athletes and World Champions in boxing, kickboxing, cross training and rugby. To my surprise they found it difficult to stay the course with me when they trained alongside me.

What seemed like an easy two to three hour workout to me, was pure pain to them. This could be due to the stamina gene and, of course, staying on top of my training, regardless of the weather conditions. To stay at the top of your field you must train in all weather conditions. This helps the body to adapt to any situation you might come across when competing, indoors or out. On some occasions when I have attempted 26-mile mountain marathons carrying 40/50 lb back packs, the weather has changed in the blink of an eye. One minute it was sunny and the next it could be heavy showers, or even snowing. This is where your all-weather training kicks in; you are prepared mentally to dig deep and stay focused. A lot of athletes are choosy and only train when they feel like it, or if it's a warm day. They will only get so far within their chosen sport.

WORLD
RECORD FEDERATION

CERTIFICATE

PADDY DOYLE

WORLD FITNESS
ENDURANCE RECORD

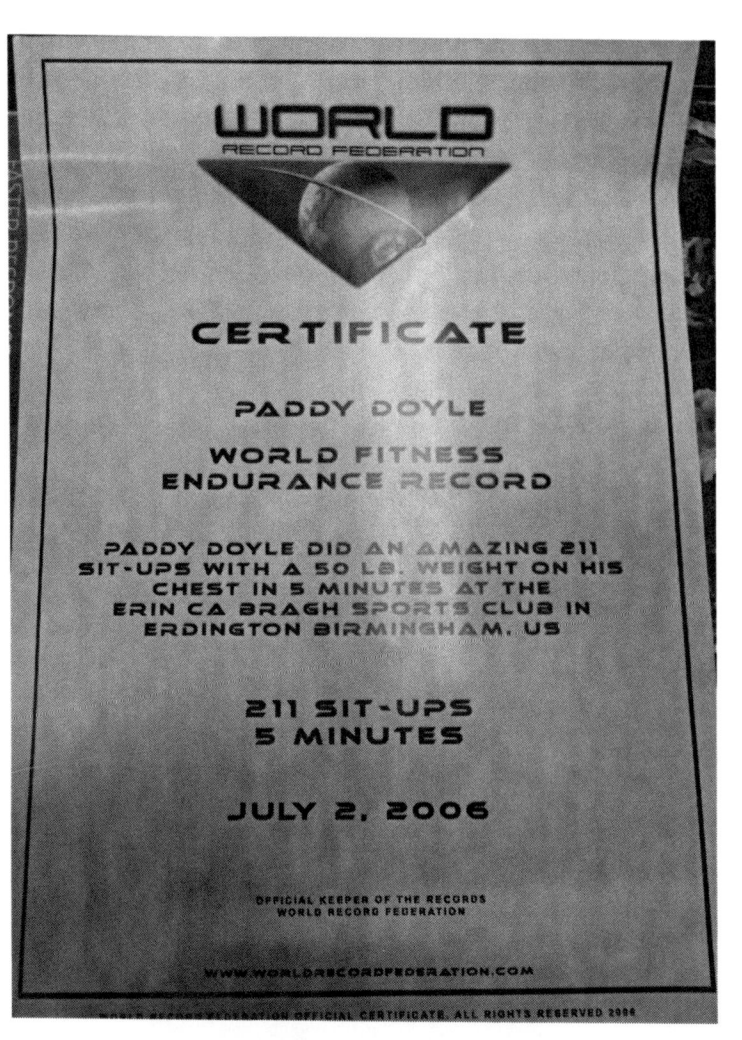

PADDY DOYLE DID AN AMAZING 211
SIT-UPS WITH A 50 LB. WEIGHT ON HIS
CHEST IN 5 MINUTES AT THE
ERIN CA BRAGH SPORTS CLUB IN
ERDINGTON BIRMINGHAM, US

211 SIT-UPS
5 MINUTES

JULY 2, 2006

OFFICIAL KEEPER OF THE RECORDS
WORLD RECORD FEDERATION

WWW.WORLDRECORDFEDERATION.COM

{most strength sit ups in 5 minutes}

Joe Egan, Former heavyweight Professional Boxer, and Mike Tyson's sparring partner said:

'Paddy Doyle is a man amongst men. He is truly a great all- round athlete and a man I am very proud to call my friend. Whilst I was a sparring partner to Mike Tyson I went through a lot of pain barriers but how Paddy Doyle pushes himself through so many pain barriers is beyond me! I think a machine would struggle to do what Paddy has done. If there was a title for the World's Super Athlete on the planet, I have no doubt he would win it.'

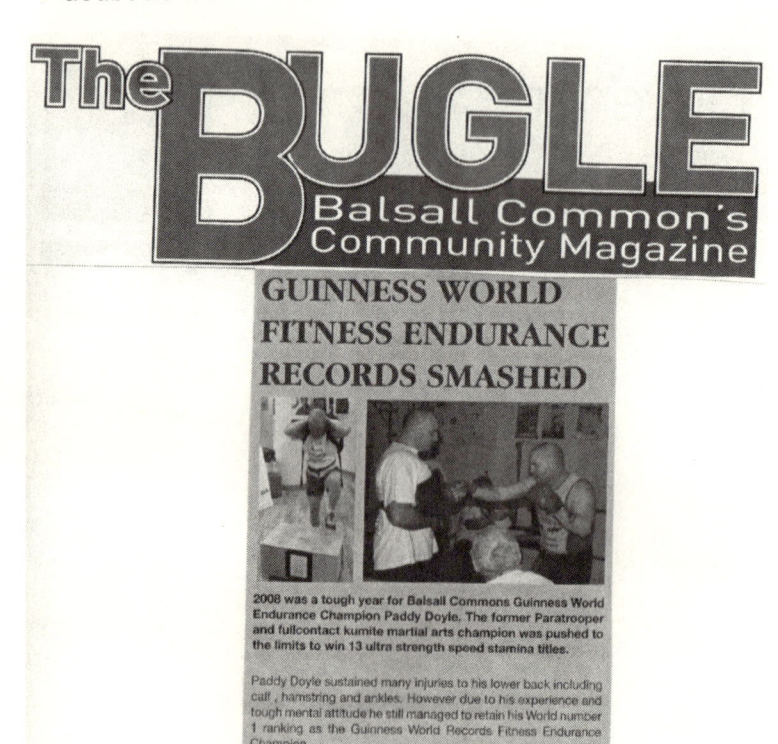

The BUGLE
Balsall Common's Community Magazine

GUINNESS WORLD FITNESS ENDURANCE RECORDS SMASHED

2008 was a tough year for Balsall Commons Guinness World Endurance Champion Paddy Doyle. The former Paratrooper and fullcontact kumite martial arts champion was pushed to the limits to win 13 ultra strength speed stamina titles.

Paddy Doyle sustained many injuries to his lower back including calf, hamstring and ankles. However due to his experience and tough mental attitude he still managed to retain his World number 1 ranking as the Guinness World Records Fitness Endurance Champion.

{Achieved 13 demanding strength speed stamina endurance records throughout 2008}

STAMINA'S GYM

I have had my gym premises for over fifteen years. It is my main base to prepare and train religiously for all of the Fitness Endurance records I have achieved to date. As you walk in the door you can smell damp and sweat. The roof leaks when it rains and when you want a shower, after pushing your body hard, you can expect a cold one. The gym equipment is made up of basic raw materials such as large truck tyres weighted down with metal plates and bricks. My students and I use the weighted tyres to carry when we are training. They weigh about 180lb, and are held in each hand. The gym walls and floor used to be covered in blood. After four years, I decided to clean the walls and floor as it was scaring new students away.

Sadly, my student membership is low as the training is very demanding, both mentally and physically. Many athletes who train want it easy and are scared of a genuine tough workout. I respect all of my students who stick the boxing and endurance circuits I throw at them. You cannot beat a back street gym and while it will probably not have flashy equipment, you are guaranteed a good workout and staying in shape, as well as meeting down-to-earth people. On a few occasions I have had boxers and martial artists join the club purely to challenge me. They have asked to train with me during the physical fitness sessions and then asked to spar with me in the ring.

A doorman, who was a Thai boxer and had fought in the ring, insisted on sparring with me. We entered the ring and I took my time, moving around and picking my shots at a steady level, holding back on my power. He came out in the first round throwing bombs. I covered up, thinking he wanted to knock me out. Paul Jones shouted time. The second round began and I went out and stepped up the power, throwing punches and kicks to his head and body. By the end of the second round he'd had enough. He was battered and bruised. He declined to come out for the third round and after that rumble in the ring, he was a lot more respectful to me.

Unfortunately he never came back to the gym again. Shortly afterwards, there was another incident. A former soldier started coming to the gym. He had also boxed at a good level, but sadly became involved in drug dealing. He was fast with his hands and could move around the ring. On one training evening he came into the gym shouting, 'I want to fight tonight!' I knew straight away he was on either cocaine or some hyper drug. After the endurance training he asked me to spar with him. I put the gloves on, thinking it was going to be a war.

The first round started and he came out like a stick of dynamite, throwing powerful fast shots. I thought, 'Fuck this,' and let rip, breaking his nose. There was blood everywhere. It calmed him down and at the end of the round he thought it was over. I said, 'Let's go another round.' His eyes widened and he looked a bit shocked. My reason for suggesting this was because he had shown disrespect and I wanted to teach him a lesson. The second round came and I pummelled him all over the ring, bruising his face and ribs. It certainly knocked the chip off his shoulder, as he was also known to use knuckle-dusters in street brawls. Men like that, in my eyes, are cowards and someone has to sort them out. I was pleased that Stamina's Gym had achieved that. I never saw him again. Later I was informed that he had been imprisoned for biting a doorman's ear off, selling drugs, and armed robbery.

The students who attend the club training sessions know very well what is expected of them. We train hard and fight hard. On one occasion I was sparring with one of my training partners, Wayne Bernstein, who at that time was a sergeant in the West Midlands Police Force. Wayne was a strong puncher and had a solid chin. I knew I had to slightly increase my power to keep away from his left hooks… if they caught me I would know about it. I countered his punch and he accidentally head- butted my straight left jab which unfortunately broke his nose. I could see that the bone had snapped and blood was pouring everywhere.

His blood was making a mess of my boxing ring mats, which was pissing me off, plus he had bruised my knuckles. He went in to work the next day, and from what he told me, the senior Police Inspector was not very happy and wanted to know what had been going on. Wayne told the Police Inspector that a fellow police officer had done it whilst they were training. I have known Wayne for many years. We are always winding each other up. I suppose my way of winding him up was by breaking his nose. Well, that's what friends are for…

Sean Blyth, President of the World Gym Challenge, 2007:

'I met Paddy Doyle in the last few days of spring 2007, travelling up from Kent to Birmingham to train at his gym, the Erin Go Bragh Sports Centre. I was unsure how to react when I first met him. I had recently read his autobiography which he he'd signed and sent me. I knew he was a tough cookie (his titles speak for themselves), but I needn't have worried. He shook my hand warmly, introduced me to his students and treated me with the utmost respect whilst I was there. Meeting Paddy has been a highlight. I am satisfied with what makes people endure pain and how they tolerate their pain levels, when others quit. The mind plays such a vital role in preparation; that counts for so much. At the end of the day, you have to get through barriers, finish, and live to tell the tale. Paddy does that.

'At Paddy's Gym you start from scratch. Paddy isn't interested what you have on your feet, what top you wear, or if you have shaved. He is interested in getting you to train and work hard. It's never a popular class – nor, I suspect, will it ever be. Paddy gets you to work. He tells you to do something and you do it, as much as it hurts at that time, and you don't want to let him down. You need to have a certain persona to make people perform, but at the same time, you have to be the right type of person to endure Paddy's training. The reason why I said it will never be a popular class is quite simply that it is hard work and most gyms today won't embrace this type of hard workout. But I'll tell you this, I trained with Paddy Doyle for one night. I will remember it for a lifetime, as will all the guys who train with him. I will go back to my gym for the rest of my days there, knowing what hard training is all about, and that will have nothing to do with the plasma screens, the air conditioning, the fresh plants, or the receptionists. It will have to do with Erin Go Bragh Sports Centre and Paddy Doyle. I ached for three days afterwards.'

GUINNESS WORLD RECORDS DAY

November 13th 2008 was another big day for me. I was attempting to set a new 30-mile cross country record carrying a 40lb back pack on the Arden Warwickshire Challenge walk, and also beat a separate record which was 10km carrying a 40lb pack, a record which was held by Robin Simpson (Leeds). My support team were great. I decided to go for the 10km speed march record first. I had to beat 57 mins 31 secs. The officials counted me down and I was off. I had to sprint as fast as I could. The weather conditions were ideal, no wind or rain. I knew that if I could maintain the speed, the record was within my grasp. Brian Vernum, one of the team members, was shouting at me to keep going. I started to get blisters at the seventh mile; my feet were feeling the impact from the tarmac.

At last I could see the finishing line and made one last sprint. The official time was 57 mins: 2 secs. I knew I had very little time to spare as the support team and I had to make our way to the Arden 30-mile start line at Henley-in-Arden, Warwickshire. I managed to eat some bananas and get a hot drink. The weather was starting to break as heavy rain and wind built up.

The countdown came and I was off. My tactic was to gain as much ground as possible, the reason being I knew the footpaths and hills would get worse as the day went by.

My worst nightmare came true, for the path leading up to Banhams Wood was terrible. Once again I was taking two steps forward and four steps back. What also did not help was that the blisters from the previous World Record challenge that morning, had started to burst open. As the miles went by the rain made the route more difficult. I was slipping on the mud, and my lower back and knees were also feeling the strain of the back pack and cold weather. I was pleased to reach each check point, as this gave me enough time to fuel up, change my clothing and get back on track. The final stage of the walk was over the slippery Arden Golf course.

I was starting to feel it at that stage. Besides my injuries, I was feeling dizzy and light-headed but my pacer, Stewart Mitchinson, a Detective Constable from West Mercia Police, and John Court, former ABA boxing coach, kept me going to the finishing line. Had Stewart not been there on the last few miles with me, I believe I would have sat down and rested, thereby losing valuable time and possibly getting hypothermia. At last I could see the team waiting at the finish line. I was relieved and pleased it was all behind me. My body was aching all over and the cold was getting to me. I have to admit on this occasion that the cold and the weight of the back pack made me feel sick, tired and mentally drained. My finishing was time was 7 hrs, 52 mins, 23 secs, setting a new cross-country record.

Once I got into the house I lay in the bath for an hour, resting my body and thinking about the tough day I had completed.

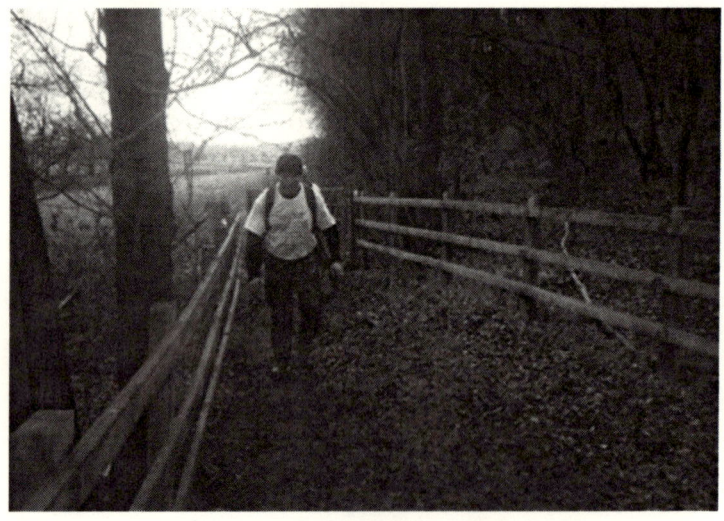

{ Arden cross country Coughton checkpoint start}

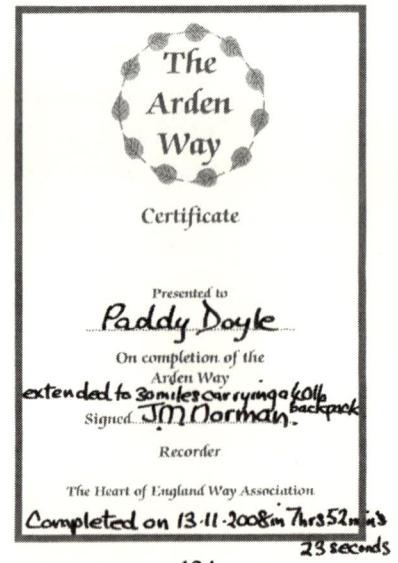

The Arden Way

Certificate

Presented to

Paddy Doyle

On completion of the
Arden Way extended to 30 miles carrying a 60lb backpack
Signed... JM Norman.

Recorder

The Heart of England Way Association

Completed on 13·11·2008 in 7hrs 52mins 23 seconds

CHALLENGERS AND JEALOUS TALKERS

A year ago, a cross training champion who was ranked third in the country, a former Marine, bad-mouthed me over the phone. I spoke to him, saying you never make assumptions about anyone, especially if you have never met them. He paused and apologised. I invited him to my gym for a workout and a sparring session. He made some excuses saying he had a bad back and a glass jaw. I found this very confusing as he had stated that he boxed for the Marines. I rang him three more times but he kept saying he was busy. I did say to him that I could get him picked up from his home and dropped back, but he still declined. I will let you, the readers, decide about that one...

More recently, a British endurance athlete from Leeds, UK, has been saying he is going to take all of my fitness endurance records off me. Most annoying is that some of his training partners have been sending me childish, jealous emails. But as I have always said, I do not hide behind computers, so I managed to get hold of their mobile numbers and rang them direct. I asked them what the problem was. Their replies were weak and full of bullshit. Basically, they could not answer my questions and were surprised that I had their mobile numbers. I did invite them down to my gym to train with me as they were stating on the internet how good they are at fitness and martial arts, but to date they have not shown their faces. They know who they are. I also texted them my mobile number with a message saying any problems or issues, ring me.

When I was in the USA representing Great Britain at the World Record Breakers Cup Challenge, I was hoping to see my arch rival, James Clarke. He had beaten some of my strength sit-ups records with a 50lb weight on the chest. He was another one who told an American newspaper that he was going to take more of my records off me. When I turned up at the venue at Coney Island he was not there. I told the senior Adjudicator, Dr David Adamovich, that I would have liked to meet and challenge James Clarke, but no more was said. I suppose when you are at the top, you will come across individuals who want to knock you down. My approach is to confront them there and then and nip things in the bud.

For the last two years I have been training my students to achieve World Records under the strength speed stamina category. To date they have set and broken a total of twelve fitness endurance records. I get great pleasure from seeing other athletes benefit from my coaching, knowledge and experience. I am training a new breed of endurance athletes who come from established sports, such as amateur boxing, karate, running, long distance walking and rugby. I strongly believe that you should pass on your skills to those who want to learn, and so far I am having great success.

I never thought that one day I would be training your average Joe Bloggs at my gym, and getting him to achieve a British, World or Masters physical fitness record. I am so proud of them when they achieve their goals. The year 2008 was a tough one for me, setting and breaking World Records. I have achieved ten more fitness endurance records, picking up a lot of injuries along the way, such as a cut hand which needed stitches. That accident happened when I was training for the four fitness endurance records on 13 May 2008. I was speed marching over fields and hills carrying a 50lb back pack and decided to take a short cut over a barbed wire fence, but as I jumped the fence my hand got caught on the barbed wire and ripped some flesh from the palm of my hand.

PUSHING IT TO THE LIMITS

This is a subject I have always avoided in my mind, but I knew there were consequences for me after attempting the ultra physical fitness records which lasted for 24 hours or more. It has taken many years for me to realise that pushing your body and mind to the extreme can sometimes affect your line of thought. When you train hard day and night preparing for ultra fitness World Records, and when you have achieved beating it on the day, it does have its side effects. I have suffered from aggressive mood swings, hyperventilation and feeling lonely. These, I suppose, are a few of the side effects an endurance athlete has to go through, especially when he is attempting tough endurance boxing martial arts challenges. What a lot of people don't understand is that I have been pushing my body constantly at extreme fitness levels for twenty years, beating some of the world's hardest physical fitness challenges out there, under several different sporting categories.

I have also suffered many injuries, but that is part of the process of wanting to be the best. Really, the injuries are not worth moaning about. But pushing your body until it wants to break, and then your mind telling you to ignore the consequences, is bound to produce mental scars. To what extent, I will probably find out in the future. My advice to all endurance athletes is be prepared, as it is a lonely road. You have to be selfish and sometimes, relationships have to come second. Your training comes first and nothing else. Would I do it all over again?' My answer is yes... I would.

There was another tough record challenge which stood out. The para jumps (burpees). This exercise is a combination between a squat and squat thrust. It puts a lot of pressure on your lower back, hamstrings, calves, triceps and shoulders. I decided to go for a para jumps endurance record averaging 3000/4000 per day for seven days. On the last day I had to complete 3000, finishing on a final total of 21,409. What was different about this record was that my team was carrying out a scientific test. I was wearing a heart rate monitor, which later produced some amazing results. Of all days, it happened to be one of the hottest days of the year when the World Record took place at the Royal International Air Tattoo, Fairford. At that time I was a serving RAF Reservist Soldier and was asked to represent my Squadron by attempting a fitness endurance record. Which I was honoured to do. My support team was John Williams, osteopath; Peter Taylor, sports therapist; and Frank Daly who paced me at various stages of the three-hour finale.

I remember the sun beating down on the back of my neck and legs. Cramp had also started to kick into my legs, but I would not give in or stop. Frank was pushing me hard to keep the pace going. I stopped every 100 repetitions for a quick drink of water and carried on. Due to the constant heat, the last two hundred repetitions were a blur. The sweat and salt was burning my eyes and all I could hear was, 'STOP!' John Williams said, 'Paddy, you've done it.'

I was so pleased it was over. My neck and legs were blistered from the sun and my eyes were sore from the salt and sweat which I had endured for the last three hours.

John Williams, Osteopath/Physiotherapist 2009, had this to say:

'With a keen interest in sport and fitness, I was fascinated by the physiology of Paddy's body. His fitness and endurance feats make him stand out from others and I wanted to know what makes him so special and mentally tough. Anyone who has met Paddy soon realizes he has an abundance of mental strength and sheer determination with a 'never quit' attitude, but that alone could not achieve the success of his previous records. Many people can 'talk the talk' but few can 'walk the walk.'

'I was particularly interested in a more scientific approach to this World Record. I introduced a heart rate monitor which was to be worn by Paddy during the challenge. This particular exercise usually sends the heart rate soaring and fatigue usually follows very quickly. We were to take readings at every minute and the results would be recorded at the end of the record attempt. My physiotherapy colleague, Peter Taylor, agreed to assist with recording the data.

'The World Record was to be outside on a staged

platform with no protection from the sun. The temperature on the tarmac must have been in the 80's with no protection whatsoever. Spectators were sweating and I was concerned about dehydration, as it was to be a long event. It was decided that after every 100 para jumps, or burpees, Paddy would stop for a drink of water, and at 500 para jumps he would have a two minute rest break and rub down. After the first hour I could not believe the results that were being recorded for his heart rate. Paddy's heart was steadily up to 130bpm and maintained this level continuously, to within 3 beats, throughout the challenge. The pattern was similar throughout the day, and this reading would be equivalent to someone jogging.

Another amazing observation was that Paddy never pulled even one short repetition as part of the challenge. He had observers watching for flawed technique and every single para jump was strict. This is incredible when you see tiredness creeping in and still Paddy maintains the discipline to deliver technically perfect para jumps. All I can say is, well done, we are all very proud of him and honoured to be a part of it all.'

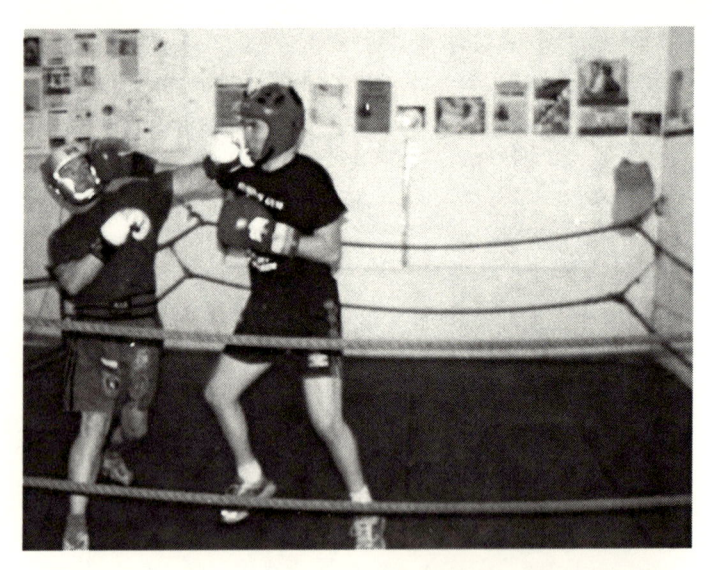

{Intense full contact sparring training for World Record Challenge, with Hard Hitting Matthew Petrie right of the picture against Paddy Doyle}.

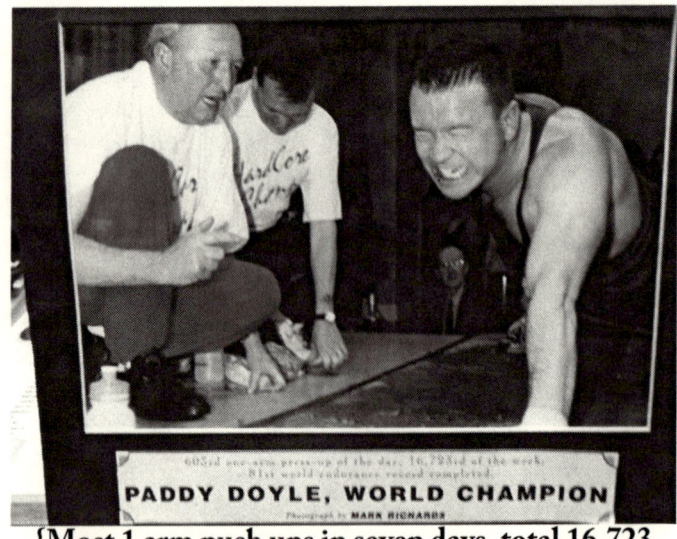

{Most 1 arm push ups in seven days, total 16,723 averaging 2,389 per day set on 18th Feb 96}

LETTING OFF STEAM

My belief has always been that if I put one hundred percent into whatever I do, then I should be allowed to chill out and let off steam. When I used to go out with my mates I always got a little bit pissed, and it could get a bit rowdy with idiots pushing you in the bars; if another bloke pushes you, then you have to push him back. On one occasion, a doorman/bouncer in a Solihull bar pushed me, which was totally out of order. I told him to fuck off and left the bar with my mates. But the incident was on my mind all week.

When Friday night came, I made my way into Birmingham and met up with my mate. We had a few drinks and moved onto the next bar where, to my surprise, I bumped into the bouncer who had pushed me the week before. I confronted him and told him he had been out of order for pushing me. I told him that I was prepared to sort it out there and then in the car park. He said he did not want any trouble with me and apologized. Although he was around 6ft 2ins and weighed around 238lbs, I was ready to have a straightener there and then.

When I was in the Parachute Regiment, I sometimes went off the rails, getting pissed and into fights with soldiers from other Regiments. One Saturday night

I went with another Para to the local chip shop. We were making our way back to the barracks when some soldiers on the other side of the road shouted at us, saying we were no good. I went over to speak to them politely. One of them threw a punch which struck me on the shoulder. I then hit him back, putting him on his arse. At almost the same moment, the Military Police pulled up and jumped on me. I was escorted back to Bruneval Barracks and once again put in jail. I was kicking myself as I knew I was in deep shit. I would rather have been in a civilian prison than an army jail. I was marched in front of the Commanding Officer the next morning, and told that I would lose my pay and privileges and do extra Physical Fitness Training for a month.

For the next month I had to get up at 4am every morning and clean my cell and the jail house toilets and showers with other Para prisoners. We then had to do cleaning duties around the barracks such as emptying the bins, sweeping the paths and cleaning all the pots in the cookhouse. We would sometimes get to our beds at midnight, due to all the shitty tasks which we had to do as part of our punishment. The Regimental Police also made us quick march everywhere. This was difficult as we had no laces in our boots. The reason for this was to stop us doing a runner or escaping from the camp. When you are a prisoner you are also subjected to hard, challenging, physical beatings. Whatever the weather, you were made to run, crawl and do circuit training exercises until you dropped. I have to admit it… I loved every minute of it. Although I hated being locked up in the cell, I came out a better and fitter soldier.

I remember an occasion when I was invited to Redditch for a few drinks by Gary Bernstein the twin brother of Wayne 'the nutter' Bernstein. I remember clearly that I was looking forward to a relaxing Friday night. I'd had a tough week of intensive training and wanted to get pissed, but once again that never happened.

There were six of us who met up in a local pub, minding our own business. I went up to the bar to order a round of drinks and as I was waiting to be served, a tall bloke bumped into me. He looked down at me, stared, and made some aggressive comments. I ignored him and carried on getting the drinks in. This is **Gary's** account of what happened:

'As I recall, there was a group of six of us out for a drink in Redditch. Within our group was Paddy and his friend John McBean, who was a former professional cruiserweight boxer and ex-ABA champion. Whilst we definitely were not looking for any trouble, it was fairly obvious to any half intelligent person that it would be a mistake to try and mess with us. But the bottom line is that the last thing we were looking for was a fight.

We went for a quiet drink at the Gate Hangs Well in Redditch, and there we were, minding our own business, sitting round a table enjoying a drink, and having a good chat. In the pub there was a big guy. It was clear that he was not happy... you could just tell from his body language and attitude that he was a trouble maker. For some completely unknown reason he started looking at our group, and making comments. People in the pub were giving him a wide berth, and I had the impression that he was known in the pub, but that nobody was prepared to tackle him.

As previously mentioned, the last thing that we wanted was trouble, so when this guy went to the toilet, my brother took the opportunity to have a quiet word with the people who knew him. He advised them that if he was spoiling for a fight he would be making a big mistake, and it would be in his best interests to either calm down or go home.

It was good advice that should have been taken. The problem was, I think, that this big guy thought he was quite handy with his fists, and he was probably used to people being frightened of him. We all continued to mind our own business and continue with our drinks. I recall that we were sitting on stools around the table, just chatting away.

A few minutes later, this guy approached our group and stood behind Paddy. He tapped him on the shoulder, raised his fists, and then made the monumental mistake of inviting Paddy outside for a fight. You could see that Paddy was completely calm, and he agreed to accommodate his invitation. In one swift movement, Paddy began to stand up, throwing a left hook in the process. It landed flush on the guy's jaw and he was unconscious before he even hit the floor. He should have listened and gone home.

However, there was another problem. Paddy checked up on the guy's condition while he was still spark out on the floor. He had swallowed his tongue. Once again Paddy acted swiftly. He cleared his airway and put him in the recovery position, and the guy gradually regained consciousness. When he managed to stand up, I don't think he knew who or what had hit him, but at long last he did realise it was time to go home!

The owner of the pub came over to us, and thanked Paddy. The guy had been a problem in the pub previously, but nobody had been prepared to tackle him. I have returned to the pub several times since and never seen him in there again. Perhaps he finally learnt his lesson and realised that he wasn't quite as tough as he thought he was.'

COURSES AND HOBBIES

I have always loved outdoor adventure training. A lot of my training was done in North Wales, Peak District, Lake District and the Cairngorm Mountains. I decided in 2003 to enrol on a Mountain leader Training Course with the Bremex Trust. Bremex, when it was up and running, was a hill/mountain/rock climbing training organisation. The first training weekend was under the guidance of the well known author and experienced mountain guide, Mal Creasey. Mal put us through our paces on the first day, giving us difficult navigational points to find. What did not help was the heavy constant rain, wind and cold. But that's what becoming a mountain leader is all about; you have to operate and adapt in all conditions.

I have to admit it was one of the toughest courses I have completed with regard to being mentally switched on. The fitness, although it was challenging, was never a problem. I found the theory and responsibilities of a mountain leader a lot to take on board. At that time I was training for an endurance 40lb back pack course record, so I decided foolishly to add extra weight to my back pack on the course. Although I was improving my stamina levels, I paid for it later on in the course by feeling tired and not taking on board the skills required on the mountains to become a mountain leader.

However, I was determined to pass the course. I had to put the time in as part of my log book training, so one weekend in every three to six weeks for the next three years, I travelled to North Wales attending mountain leader workshops. The reason for me wanting to take the time to put in as many training hours as possible was because I never had easy access to mountains, as I lived in central England. Whilst I was training for my Mountain Leader Award, I decided to go for the Walking Group Leader Award which enables you to take groups out in low-level hill areas. This gave me more experience and confidence working in challenging environments.

Whilst on the course I met Barry Lynn, who is now a good friend. The reason I have mentioned Barry is because he has a slight disability and cannot use his left arm properly. My admiration goes to him because he stuck at the mountain leader training and passed successfully in 2005. To me and others, that shows determination and you can achieve like Barry did, if you put your mind to it. Thankfully, I passed my Mountain Leader Award a year later in 2006, and have recently completed my Winter Mountain Leader Training in the Scottish Cairngorms, with Phill George. Phill, who is based in North Wales, is another respected mountain instructor. The winter mountain training is a serious course. I found that fitness levels had to be higher than those for the summer mountain leader. This is due to working in a more challenging environment. Phill pushed us every day, possibly testing us, to see if we were the right sort of individuals to become Winter Mountain Leaders.

I remember the morning when we stayed out in a snow hole. I was paired with Ian Ridley, who was a great partner to have on the course, as he had some previous experience of winter training. Ian was winding me up and joking with me throughout the week so I thought I would play a trick on him. When you need to go to the toilet in the mountains, you now have to poo into a large tube. The reason for this is to prevent contamination of the environment. On the morning of packing up and leaving our snow hole, I pooed in my tube, sealed it, and waited until we got back to our sleeping quarters. After our one-to-one briefings on the last day, I sneaked into Andy's bunker and put the poo into his bag. Like a good mountaineer, he took it home with him in his car. He later found it and sent me a nice polite email. I knew I would wind him up in my way.

But that's the sort of humour you need to have to be able to train and work in winter conditions of that nature. Outdoor instructors, in my opinion, have to be thicker-skinned than your normal leisure fitness instructors. Let's face it, when you are in the hills and mountains and something goes wrong you have not got a phone to run to. If the shit hits the fan, the buck… and the pressure, stops with you.

Mal Creasey, author and Mountain leader Training Technical officer, 2009:
'Well, what can I say about Paddy that has not already been said? He is currently a larger than life character which is just as well, because in fact he ain't that tall! Seriously though, he has a big heart and is a

real nice fella underneath that hard man image. From what I have seen, he is quick to jump to the defence of those less able to defend themselves and he doesn't take kindly to any injustices he comes across.

'I first met Paddy on a wet and windy Saturday afternoon in North Wales when he embarked upon a Mountain Leader training course and… I'm sure he won't mind me saying me this… during that session, it became pretty obvious that Paddy had a serious amount of work to do if he was going to be successful. Needless to say, he had the heaviest rucksack in the world (lead weights or bricks, I'm not sure which). He was training for a speed march record at that time! Well that was a few years ago and as you can imagine, Paddy being the man he is, applied himself to the tasks required with enthusiasm, dedication and hard graft. It was just another challenge and he wasn't going to be beaten! No one was more pleased than me when he qualified for the Mountain Leader Award.

'Paddy was attempting a cross country hill course record in the Staffordshire moorlands, and I was asked to attend as an official. I found myself involved with yomping (or is it tabbing?) through the Staffordshire countryside escorting high-heeled BBC radio presenters through muddy fields, which he successfully completed with his training team and ex-Parachute Regiment colleagues. You never know with Paddy what he might go for next. You can't keep a man like that down with his infectious enthusiasm. I have no doubt there will be more World Record challenges ahead, and no doubt our paths will cross again soon. I look forward to that day.'

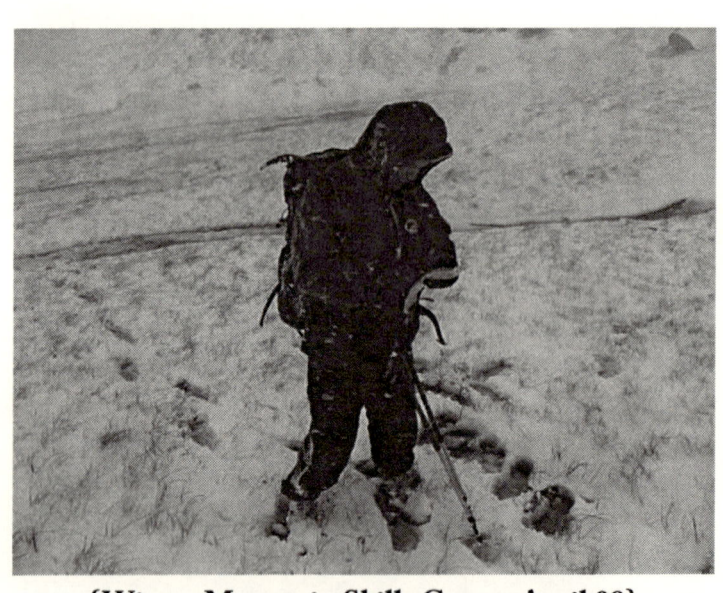

{Winter Mountain Skills Course April 09}

CONTACTS AND FRIENDS

I've got some great friends in Liverpool; it is a great city and full of characters. Joe Lynch has been very supportive and has backed me on numerous World Records. Joe owns Liverpool's number one nightclub, *Society*. He is a successful business man along with his brother John Lynch, who is a former pro boxer and boxing gym owner. Another member of the Liverpool crew who has been giving me some advice and guidance on certain matters, is Charlie Seiga. He came from a life of crime and Police once believed that he was behind armed bank robberies, wage snatches and other serious crimes, including contract beatings, but they remained unable to convict him.

I was introduced to the crew by Alan Ashes who is a former Special Forces Soldier and nightclub doorman working for Joe Lynch. I have a lot of respect for these guys as they have always made me welcome when I have met up with them in Liverpool and shown me respect. I was told of a few incidences and stories whilst on my visit, but I'm afraid I was sworn to secrecy. But it's great to get advice from them. They are all older than I am, which is why I listen to them… because they have been there and made a success of their lives from their mistakes. A lot of the lads also come from Irish backgrounds like myself; their parents came over to the UK from Ireland, just after the war. All of them came from poor backgrounds similar to mine and they have also worked their way up in life.

I have learnt throughout my life that you have to surround yourself with genuine characters from all walks of life, and when the shit hits the fan it's good to seek advice from those who have learnt the hard way themselves. On those occasions when I have been in trouble, or had confrontations with bullies and idiots, my friend Big David Chubb has always stood by me, given me advice and calmed me down. If it had not been for David when I had that fight in the bar in Germany, I could have been locked up in a German prison cell. I have to admit it, I was enjoying punching the hell out of the big German who was aggressive towards me in the bar. However, it could have got serious as I wanted to destroy him, but David walked in and stopped me.

I owe a lot to David and also his partner, Kerry. They arranged for me to meet Deborah, who is a close friend of Kerry's. I have been with Deborah for over three years now and we are going strong. We recently got engaged in New York, after I had attempted the one minute back-of-hands push-ups records and I do feel very happy and content. She has brought me stability and I love her to bits.

Sponsorship has been hard to come by, but one man who has backed me for the last eighteen months is Jim Mosley of Co-op Construction Ltd. His company is a pay roll accountancy business and without his backing I would have retired long ago. In the earlier part of my athletic career Tony and Maggie Ryan of MarCity

Developments, Solihull, were also a great support in sponsoring me for Guinness World Records. I had the pleasure of training Tony Ryan, helping him to prepare for the London Marathon in 2005 in which he raised £30,000 for his chosen charity. I paced him for the length of the 26 mile course. I remember when we got to the finish line how proud I was of him, as he had gone through a tough time in preparing for the event. What people didn't realise was that he was 6ft 5ins tall and weighed 18 stones.

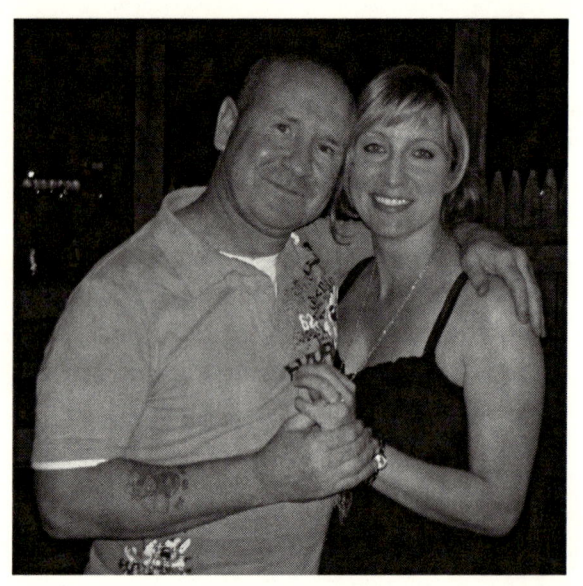

{Paddy and Deborah getting engaged in New York August 2008}

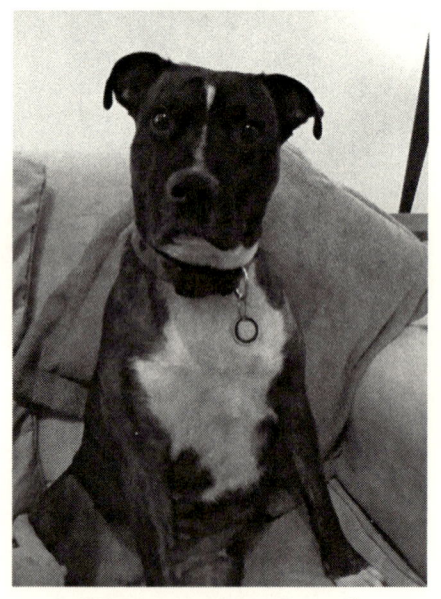

{Trixie my best friend}

DOYLE'S WORLD RECORD TOTAL FITNESS TRAINING PREPARATION TIPS

Many athletes, coaches and members of the general public have asked me how do I train and prepare to achieve such incredible feats of endurance. I will now give a breakdown of my training methods which I hope everyone will be able to use within their own fitness workouts. Since attempting my first fitness endurance record in May 1987, and still pushing my body to the extreme twenty-one years later, I have learnt a lot about myself both mentally and physically. This self-knowledge has helped me to break a career total of 170 strength fitness endurance records which cover several different sporting disciplines. I would like to share some of this knowledge with you, the readers, so you can benefit in much the same way as I have.

Before I start a training workout I will mentally prepare myself with the personal goals I intend to achieve during the workout. Usually this will involve doing more repetitions at a faster pace, and adding further exercises to my programme. The important point is that I always aim to improve on my previous training workout. I believe all male/female athletes and average persons wishing to improve their fitness levels can do the same to achieve a good standard of competitive fitness levels.

The exercise programmes, health advice and nutrition I have outlined in this programme have a multitude of benefits to sportsmen and women as well as those wishing to reach and maintain a good standard of fitness. I have tried to describe the following facts and tips in a simple bullet point format. Now read on… and I'll show you the steps I took to become a Guinness World Records Multi Fitness Endurance Champion.

World Record Workout

My training schedule would depend on what multi-fitness endurance record or martial arts-boxing challenge I would attempt to go for. If, for example, it would be a back pack speed march over the Welsh Mountains, I would speed march on Mondays, Wednesdays and Fridays with a back pack weighing a lot heavier than the weight I would be carrying on the day of the challenge. I would be training with a 70lb pack which would benefit me by strengthening my legs and improving my stamina. The standard World Record weight is 40lb when attempting any recognized World Record distance. Even I have regular medical check ups by my Doctor to ensure that my body can cope with the intense training. My advice to anyone participating in any form of exercise, especially if you have not trained for some time, is to have a medical check up with your own Doctor.

World Record Training Programme Endurance Speed March Back Pack Records

1. Monday. Speed march with back pack 70lb.
2. Tuesday. Running without back pack distance 6-7 miles, 20 mins circuit training distance 5 miles, 3 rounds on punch bag, 4 x 3mins rounds on punch bag, pad work, 25mins circuit training, 4 rounds full contact sparring.
3. Wednesday. Speed march with back pack 5 miles.
4. Thursday. Running 4 miles, 10mins circuit training, 15mins non stop circuit training, 2 rounds bag work, 4 rounds full contact martial arts sparring, 3 rounds full contact martial arts boxing sparring, 5 miles gym cycle, 10,000 metres rowing.
5. Friday. Speed march with back pack 10 miles, 15mins circuit training, 2 rounds punch bag, 3 rounds full contact martial arts boxing sparring.
6. Saturday. Rest.
7. Sunday. Swim 20-30 lengths, slow run 3 miles.

Comments and Bullet Point Facts

As you can see, each training day varies. It is essential that I use a cross training section of endurance routines as it will enhance my all-round performance. Sticking to the same workout could put a lot of strain on my body, and would do the same to other athletes wishing to use the same training methods.

I stopped regular running about five years ago and started uphill mountain walking. It was the best thing I had done. The pain to my knees and lower back were reduced, the reason being that there was less impact to my joints, plus I was learning navigational skills which it made it more interesting. It is fact that when you run, the impact of a running step can be three to four times your own body weight, whilst walking is only one and a half times. The benefits of walking, whether it be on flat ground or on the hills, are:

- Burns as many calories as running/jogging.
- Less stress to your joints.
- Improves stamina levels.
- Lowers blood pressure.
- Reduces your waist line.
- Is an excellent way of reducing stress.
- Tones muscles.
- Improves your cardio/aerobic levels.

My advice for anyone wishing to start uphill walking as part of their training workout is as follows:

- Complete 20 to 30 step-ups carrying 10/20lb dumbbells. This builds up your quad muscles which strengthens your legs for the hills.
- When walking, carry a back pack which can be filled with sand weighing 10/15lb. This helps to improve your stamina and at the same time accustoms you to carrying a back pack, especially if you

are going over long hilly distances.
- To enjoy your walking training, good posture is essential. Always try and keep your back straight and relax your arms, which helps your breathing.
- Buy the right kit. Boots and walking socks are very important. Make sure they are of a reputable make, as these can reduce blisters and discomfort.
- Food intake is essential. If you are going for a 4 to 5 hour walk, you will burn up a lot of calories so you will need to have with you in your back pack: energy bars, a hot drink and some cold water, chocolate, wholemeal bread sandwiches with either tuna or cheese filling, and some nuts.

World Record Training Preparation Programme
Boxing – Martial Arts Kumite Challenge Records

When preparing for a World United Martial Arts Association Kumite Martial Arts boxing title record, I would follow the training workout with my training team and coach:

- Shadow boxing 4 x 4min rounds, rest for 30secs. Shadow boxing is excellent for stretching, improving speed and technique.
- Bag work 4 x 4min rounds. Helps with stamina,

power and skill.
- Pad work 4 x 4 min rounds. Improves co-ordination and improving combinations.
- Skipping 4 x 4min rounds. Excellent for stamina, good for footwork. Similar to running on the spot.

At the end of the session my training team and I will finish off with a fast and hard non-stop circuit training session consisting of:

- 50 push ups.
- 200 sit up crunches.
- 50 squat thrusts.
- 100 para burpees.
- 100 squats.
- 200 alternative squat thrusts.
- 10 mins static wall sit.

Repeat session.

Comments

Depending on how well the training went and if my body did not pick up any injuries, I would always increase my repetitions by an extra 40 to 50. But as you gain more experience, you learn to listen to your body. So if you feel an ache in your legs or upper body, stop, assess and stretch, and if you feel okay, then push your body further.

Ronnie Christopher, achieved a career 27 National European World Karate Title's, 2009. 'had this to say: I remember taking the Karate team down to train with Paddy to improve our squad fitness.

However Paddy's idea of fitness training was different from mine, it included getting into the ring with him and doing some full contact sparring rounds. Whilst fighting he punched me so hard in the ear, I could not hear properly for a month, he also detached the retina of another black belt team member! It was an eye opening experience and thoroughly enjoyable. My squad commented that they could not believe the intensity in how Paddy trained, they found him an inspiration. Paddy is uncompromising, both on himself and his students. He is fully committed in everything he does and his attitude has remained the same throughout these years, training is important to him and should always be done with nothing less than 100%.

'The first time I met Paddy was an experience in itself! I walked into his gym to find tall big black guys, all of them 6 foot plus of muscle, being shouted at by this stocky smaller white guy! They all listened to him and followed his instructions to the letter, such was the respect he commands from his students. He does not ask anyone to do anything that he has not done himself, he is a man who leads by example.'

Guinness Martial Arts Kumite Karate Boxing Record

Since August 2007 I have been increasing my fullcontact rounds at various martial arts clubs and WUMA kumite sanctioned events. The aim was to beat the Guinness Record for the most amateur freestyle fullcontact karate boxing rounds fought. The record I set was 6,264 fighting rounds from 15th Febuary 1993 to 7th December 2005, so on April 2nd I decided to complete the tough challenge finishing with a total of 52 rounds bringing the final total to 6,316 rounds over a sixteen year period. My hat goes off to the martial artists and boxers who gave me a hard bruising contest, the age range of each fighter was 24 yrs to 33 yrs of age. The first round was with George Dyer an excellent thai boxing martial artist, he had a long straight jab and was out reaching me with most of his punches, I knew I had to use my hooks as I was the smaller guy, the rounds seemed to be lasting long which I put down to my stamina and recent back injury.

The rounds finished and the score was I won on my points, however I thought it was close. I carried on fighting three other excellent martial artists drawing with two and losing one. Fighting with Carl Brown was the best three rounds of the night at one stage I remember taking numerous punches in our exchange, all I could to do was cover up and wait for an opening, my head cleared, I threw hooks to his head and straight jabs to his body wearing him down in the later rounds. One of the officials commented after the contest's that it was close and that I took a lot of head punches.

I was carrying an extra stone in weight which effected my performance, the excess weight was like carrying a bergen on my stomach. My face was a mess with minor cuts to my forehead, face, a bruised head, arms and ribs. But I thoroughly enjoyed the finale to the challenge. It certainly taught me a lesson to prepare better and make sure my injuries must be cleared up, but I love a hard tough challenge, however that is no excuse, at the end of the day I chose to get in their and fight.

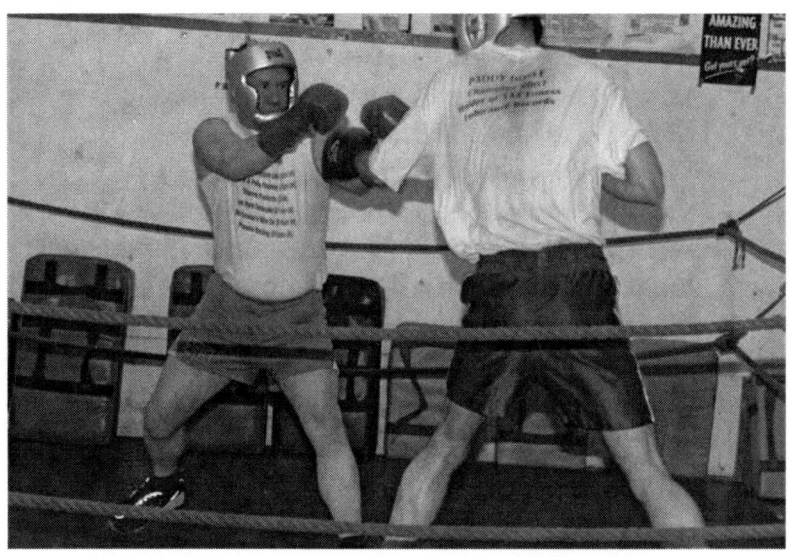

{Most Inter - Club Full contact Boxing Martial Arts Rounds Fought April 2 2009. Final Total 6,316 rounds from 15th Feb 1993 - 2 April 2009}

World Record Circuit Training Workout

When I am training for a specific fitness endurance record such as press-ups, sit-ups or para jump 'burpees,' I try and stick to the following training session.

Workout Sets

- Press-ups non-stop 40 reps. Rest for 15 secs.
- Sit-ups non-stop 100 reps. Rest for 15 secs.
- Squats non-stop 100 reps. Rest for 15 secs
- Squat thrusts non-stop 100 reps. Rest for 15 secs.
- Para Jumps (burpees) 100 reps. Rest for 15 secs.
- Static wall sit 15 mins. Rest and stretch for 1 min.
- Shuttle sprints 30ft carrying 40lb dumbbells, sets of 20. Rest and stretch for 1 min, then continue.

Comments

With this workout, depending on your progression, you can repeat the same session up to three times more. However, to reach that level, you have to make sure your body can handle it, and is properly warmed up, plus all of your mind is focused.

If the session was too easy for me, I did one of the following:

1. Cut down the rest interval between exercises from say 15 secs to 10 secs.
2. Cut down the rest interval between sets from 2 mins to 1 min.

As you progress from some of the workouts I have

mentioned, try to vary your exercise routine. This will help to retain your fitness levels, and will help you to continue to develop and see the results as your body contends with different challenges and demands. Remember to update your goals regularly to reflect your higher levels of strength, speed and stamina.

Useful tips I use before attempting a World Record are:

1. Make sure you eat something light two hours before you compete. A light carbohydrate snack such as a banana or energy bar is ideal.
2. Drink plenty of fluids before, during and after the World Record – preferably water.
3. Go for variety. All-round fitness is gained by participating in different physical fitness challenges.
4. Start slowly and build up gradually – too much, too soon can really put you off and injuries could occur.
5. Exercise with a training partner or training team – it is more challenging and it will be harder to quit if it means letting someone down.
6. Last but not least, enjoy your training. Yes, it must be challenging, but not a chore.

My Nutrition for a World Record Challenge

You must eat good wholesome food and supplements if you are to be a successful athlete in any sport. Endurance athletes need adequate supplies of complex carbohydrates, vitamins and minerals, especially potassium and other multivitamins. As a non-meat-eater, I now eat a lot of vegetarian dishes with corn meat, which has helped me to lose weight. Listed below are some of my favourite foods, the supplements I take, and the reasons for taking them.

- •PROTEIN: Represents about 15-20 % of my diet and includes corn meat, chicken and fish.
- •CARBOHYDRATES: Represents around 55-60 % of my diet and consists of potatoes, rice, pasta and plenty of vegetables.
- •FAT: Represents about 20-25% of my diet and is mainly from olive oil. Some of you may feel that my fat intake is a little high, although I would argue that as it is very calorie-dense and rich in fat-soluble vitamins, it plays an important role in the endurance athlete's diet.
- •SUPPLEMENTS: I take liver tablets and ginseng for stamina, halibut oil capsules for my joints and tendons and I take extra potassium tablets because this mineral is lost during heavy training, particularly in hot weather.
- •TREATS: I am a great believer that if you train very hard you are allowed to treat yourself. I sometimes eat chocolate bars, fish and chips, Chinese meals/ takeaways and a few beers. As long as you know you have the discipline to work it off, then spoil yourself in moderation.

Nutritional Tips

- Drinking Water. When I do a lot of exercise, it's important that I keep myself hydrated. If I am feeling thirsty, that can be sign that I am suffering. I regularly take short sips of water every 10 to 15 minutes during my workouts. Never gulp down water as it can repeat, sometimes making you feel sick.
- Training Breakfast. Never miss breakfast. A lot of athletes think it's a way of losing weight. I always eat carbs, which can be oat-based cereals. This gives me a slow release of energy and stops me wanting a mid-morning snack.
- Evening Meal. As an example I would eat vegetarian corn meat with rice salad and low fat cooking sauces. Vegetarian dishes such as lasagne and spaghetti Bolognese are all low in fat content.
- Eating After Training: When I've had a tough workout I leave it for about twenty minutes to re-charge myself, and then I eat tuna, salmon, jacket potatoes with cheese or beans and pasta. This helps to repair any torn muscle tissues which have been damaged during my workouts.
- Fat-loss Tips: Try low fat yoghurt with a banana and a glass of water. The low fat yoghurt has whey protein which helps muscles to repair. The protein can also stop you feeling hungry. Bananas provide small amounts of carbohydrate energy to kick start you and water prevents dehydration.

- **Diets:** I have personally found that certain diets (not all), are not the way to lose weight. From my point of view, if you cut out calories and certain foods, your body can lose muscle power and stamina.
- **Muscle and Power:** If you want to increase your strength and muscle, the right sort of proteins are fish, dairy products and reputable protein drinks.
- **Not All Fats Are Bad For You:** Fats which are ideal for you would be avocado, oily fish and nuts. These contribute towards a healthy heart and strong muscle tissue. Avoid saturated fats which are found in processed meals.
- **Fitness Related Circulation Problems:** When I get muscle stiffness or cramp I always eat bananas which contains potassium. This has had a great effect on reducing cramp to my legs and arms. Other remedies I have taken and would recommend are garlic, onions, fresh fruit, vegetables, oily fish and low fat dairy products. Two to three portions of fish throughout the week is ideal. Why? Because fish contains Omega 3 which is good for the heart and brain cells. It also can reduce inflammation around the joints.

The Total Fitness World Record Training programme I designed is simple and not complicated. It improves my levels of fitness when I am preparing myself for physical fitness challenges. I am always ready to modify, improve, or add new exercises to my workouts. Sports Science is developing every day and I believe if you want to be the best you must be prepared to learn new skills and techniques to advance yourself. When I train, whether it be in the gym or in the outdoor environment, I will always try and improve in one area, such as speed and number of repetitions.

A method I always use is to decrease my rest intervals at each session and at the same time increase my number of repetitions or sets. This improves my stamina levels for whatever endurance challenge I go for. I hope the information I have given, although it is only basic, will give you an idea of my daily food intake. The rest is mental strength and being blessed with the stamina gene. One final point… I do not take steroids. I believe the mind is far more powerful than any drug or steroid can ever be. Remember my motto and you will become the best there is in your chosen sport… ***No Drugs… just the Will to Win.***

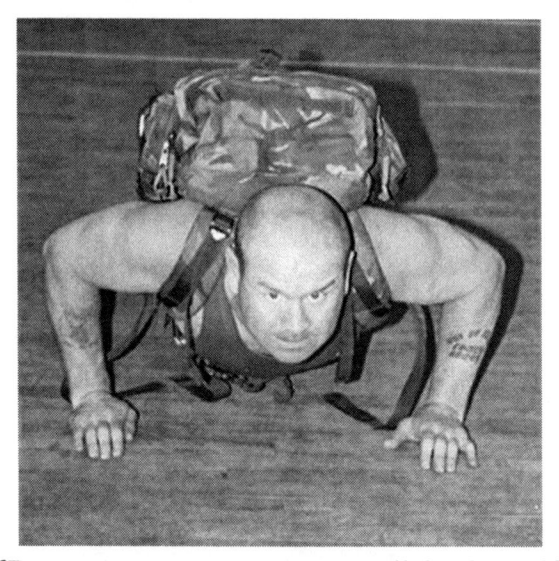

{Press ups training carrying 50 lb back pack}

Guinness Toughest World Strength Speed Stamina Records Achieved 1987 - 2008

Many individuals have asked me which World Records I have found to be the toughest. To be honest, every one of them has been hard, but the ultra-fitness records like the World Fitness Champions Record, World Ultra Cross Training Record and the Guinness Physical Fitness Challenge Record, all feats of strength, speed and stamina events, have really pushed my mind and body to the maximum. The time and effort I have put into preparing for them has been about three or four hours per day, depending on how well I was progressing.

I have listed, although not in strict order, all of my Guinness career feats of endurance Records, that I found to be the ultimate of back-breakers. The following World Records were all verified by Guinness World Records, and was awarded an official Guinness World Record certificate.

(* denotes World Record broken or modified by Guinness World Records)

1. 26-mile Wolverhampton Marathon carrying 44lb back pack.
   Time: 4 hrs, 56 mins. Set 22 May 1988. UK. *

2. 26 -mile London Marathon carrying 44 lb back pack.
   Time: 4 hrs, 42 mins, 44 secs. Broken on 21 April 1991

3. Most squat thrusts in 1 hour.
   Total: 2,010. Broken 2 Sept 1989. UK.*

4. Most squat thrusts in 1 hour.
   Total: 2,150. Broken 23 Feb 1990. UK.*

5. Most one-arm push-ups in 5 hours.
   Total: 5,260. Broken 6 May 1990. UK.*

6. Most Para Jumps (burpees) in 1 hour.
   Total: 1,619. Broken 21 June 1991. UK.*

7. Fastest 1 mile run on treadmill carrying 40lb back pack.
   Time: 6 mins, 56 secs. Set 4 Sept 1991. UK.*

8. Most Para Jumps (burpees) in 1 hour.
   Total: 1,649. Broken 19 Feb 1992. UK.*

9. Fastest 1 mile run (outdoors) carrying 40lb back pack.
   Time: 5 mins, 35 secs. Set 7 March 1993. Cork, Ireland.

10. Most one-arm push-ups in 1 hour.
    Total: 1,886. Set 27 Nov 1993. UK.

11. Most Para Jumps (burpees) in 1 hour.
    Total: 1,840. Broken 6 Feb 1994. UK.

12. Multi-fitness challenge in 1 hour.
    429 one-arm push-ups in 15 mins; 323 para

jumps in 15 mins; 400 squat thrusts in 15 mins, 592 alternate squat thrusts in 15 mins.
Set 10 April 1994. UK.

13. Most competitive full contact karate boxing rounds in 7 days.
Total: 203 rounds. Set 6 Feb 1995. UK.

14. Most one-arm push-ups in 5 hours.
Total: 8,794. Set 12 Feb 1996. UK.

15. 26-mile hill cross country speed march carrying 40lb back pack.
Time: 6 hrs, 28 mins. Set 14 Oct 1996. UK.

16. Most squat thrusts in 1 hour.
Total: 3,743. Broken 4 May 1998. UK.

17. 13-mile half marathon carrying 40lb back pack.
Time: 1 hr, 58 mins. Set 20 Sept 1998. UK.*

18. Most back-of-hands push-ups in 1 hour.
Total: 660. Set 5 March 2000. UK.*

19. Guinness/WUMA Kumite Warlords fight challenge.
131 freestyle competitive rounds in 5 hours. Set 6 May 2000. UK.*

20. Most back-of-hands push-ups in 1 hour,
Total: 1,303. Broken 21 March 2001. UK.*

21. Most back-of-hands push-ups in 1 minute.
Total: 70. Set 24 June 2001. UK.*

22. Most full contact punch strikes in 1 hour.
Total: 4,104. Set 19 Aug 2001.UK.*

23. Most kumite freestyle karate boxing rounds in 3 hrs, 6 mins.
Total: 110 rounds. Broken 9 June 2002. UK.

24. Versa Climber machine most height gained carrying 40lb back pack.
3144 ft in 1 hour. Set 17 Oct 2002. UK.*

25. Most full contact martial arts kicks in 1 hour.
Total: 2,805. Broken 7 Nov 2004. Germany.*

26. Most straight arm martial arts punch strikes in 1 minute.
Total: 470. Broken 13 Aug 2005. Germany.

27. Most freestyle amateur karate boxing inter-club rounds fought.
Total: 6,264 rounds 15 Feb 1993 - 7 Dec 2005. UK. *

28. Most step-ups (15 inch bench) in 1 hour carrying 56lb back pack.
Total: 716. Set 9 Nov 2006. UK.*

29. Most full contact punch strikes in 1 hour.
Total: 18,372 punches. Broken 19 Jan 2007. UK.*

30. Most step-ups (15 inch bench) in 1 hour carrying 40lb back pack.
Total: 911. Broken 20 April 2007. USA.*

31. Most step-ups (15 inch bench) in 1 hour carrying 40lb back pack.
Total: 1,619. Broken 13 May 2008. UK.*

32. Guinness World Records Physical Fitness Challenge Record, 11 challenges:
12 mile run; 12 mile speed march carrying 25lb back pack; 1,250 push-ups; 1,250 star jumps; 3,250 sit ups; ,250 standing hip flexors (10lb weight); 110-mile cycle; 20-mile rowing; 20-mile cross trainer; 2-mile swim; weightlifting lifted 300,000lb upper body lifts only.
Completed in 18 hrs, 56 mins, 9 secs. Broken 16 Feb 2005.UK.

33. 24-hour press-ups record.
Total: 37,350 press-ups. Broken 1 May 1989. UK.

34. 12-hour press-ups record.
Total: 19,325 press-ups. Set 1 May 1989. UK

35. Most press-ups in a calendar year.
Total: 1,500, 230. Broken 1 Oct 1989

36. World United Martial Arts Association UK Kumite Challenge Record.
141 non-stop boxing martial arts rounds in 5

hours. 117 wins, 24 losses.
Broken 19 Nov 2005

37. Most back-of-hands push-ups carrying 40lb back pack in 1 hour.
Total: 663. Set 13 May 2008

38. Most full contact straight arm punches in 1 hour.
Total: 29,850 punches. Broken 21 Jan 2008

39. Most sit-ups in 5 hours with 50lb weight on chest.
Total: 5,000. Set 28 Aug 1988

40. 1-mile back pack treadmill run carrying 40lb back pack.
Time: 6 mins, 8 secs. Set 7 Dec 1991. UK

41. Static wall sit (Samson's chair).
Time: 4 hrs, 40 mins. Broken 18th April 1990. UK.*

42. Most squat thrusts in 1 hour.
Total: 2,275. Broken 20 May 1990. UK.*

43. Fastest ½-mile run on a treadmill carrying 40lb back pack.
Time: 2 mins, 58 secs. Set 19 Sept 1991. UK.

44. Fastest 1 mile run on a treadmill carrying 40lb back pack.
Time: 6 mins, 8 secs. Set 7 Dec 1991. UK.

45. Most one-arm push-ups in 5 hours.
    Total: 7,643. Broken 31 July 1990. UK.*

46. Most miles walked carrying 30lb back pack and 9lb 9oz weight in right hand only, in downward locked position.
    Distance achieved: (time not recorded) 65 miles. Broken 3 Sept 1994.*

47. Most miles walked carrying 20lb back pack and 9lb 9oz weight in right hand only, in downward pinch grip position.
    Distance achieved: (time not recorded) 77 miles, 350 yds. Broken 10 Nov 1998.*

48. Most back-of-hands push-ups in 1 hour.
    Total: 1,940. Broken 8th Nov 2007.

49. Most back-of-hands push-ups in 1 minute carrying 40lb back pack.
    Total: 22. Set 18 March 2008. UK. *

50. Most back-of-hands push-ups in 1 minute carrying 40lb back pack.
    Total: 30. Set 16th Aug 2008. USA.*

51. Most alternativesquat thrusts in 1 hour.
    Total: 2504. Set on 3 Sept 1992. UK. *

52. Most alternative squat thrusts in 1 hour.
    Total: 2,820. Set on 27 May 1995. UK.

53. Most alternative squat thrusts in 2 hours.
    Total: 4,901. Set on 27 May 1995. UK.

54. Most push ups completed with a 50 lb weight on the back in 4 hrs 30 min's..
    Total: 4,100. Set on 28 May 1987. UK.

55. Most Para Jumps {burpees} in 30 min's.
    Total: 860. Set on 15 Feb 1992.

56. Most sit ups in 1 hour with 50 lb weight on chest.
    Total: 1,130. Set on 12 Nov 1989. UK.*

57. Most Alternative squat thrusts in 5 / 10/ 15 mins.
    Total: 290 / 545/ 740. Set on 1 and 6 August 1993. UK.

58. Most freestyle full contact karate boxing rounds in 1 calendar month.
    Total: 560. Set on 21 July – 21 August 1995. UK.

59. Fastest 5 mile run carrying 56 lb back pack.
    Time: 36 min's, 49 sec's. Set on 9 May 1999. UK.

60. Most fullcontact martial kicks in 1 hour.
    Total: 5,750. Broken on 8 Nov 2007. UK.

61. Most squats in 1 hour.
    Total: 4,708. Broken on 8 Nov 2007. UK.

62. Most fullcontact martial arts kicks in 1 hour.
Total: 1,995. Set on 30 Sept 2000. UK.*

63. Most documented amateur karate martial arts boxing rounds in 1 year.
Total: 4006. Set on 15 Feb 1993 – 15 Feb 1994. UK.

64. Most Para Jumps {burpees} in 1 hour
Total: 1,822. Broken 6 Feb 1993. UK.*

65. Most shuttle sprints carrying 100 logs weighting 56 lb each {30 feet}.
Time: 21 min's, 40 sec's. Set on 31 October 1994. UK.

66. Most shuttle sprints carrying 116 lb bag of coal {25 metres}
Time: 31 min's, 32 sec's. Set on 27 July 1992. UK.

67. Most sit ups in 15 min's with 50 lb weight on chest.
Total: 427. Set on 3 August 1991. UK.*

68. Most freestyle amateur Kumite karate boxing inter club rounds fought.
Total: 5,962 documented rounds. Set from 15 Feb 93 – 20 Feb 1999. UK.*

69. Most freestyle amateur Kumite karate boxing inter club rounds fought.
Total: 6,072 documented rounds. Set from 15 Feb 93 – 2 June 2002. UK.*

70. Most freestyle amateur Kumite karate boxing inter club rounds fought.
Total: 6,316 documented rounds. Broken on 2 April 2009. UK.

71. Most miles walked carrying 10 lb concrete slab / brick in a nominted hand in a downward pinch grip position.
Distance achieved 80. 372 miles. Broken on 21 May 2009.

World Ultra Fitness Records

Also listed is a selection of ultra World Strength Speed Stamina and individual Endurance Title Records recognised by the following world record bodies:
Registry of Record Holders:
www.recordholdersrepublic.co.uk
The World Record Federation (USA):
www.worldrecordfederation.com
The International Record Holders Club (Germany):
www.recordholders.org

1. World Strength Speed Stamina Record (12 challenges):
12-mile walk carrying 25lb back pack; 12-mile run; 2-mile swim; 110-mile cycle; weights 'upper body' 312,170lb; 1,250 press-ups; 1,250 star jumps; 3,250 sit-up crunches; 20,000-metre rowing; 1,250 hip flexors '5lb weight'; 1-mile run carrying 44lb back pack; 3-km on gym stepper; 2-mile swim.

Time: 21 hrs, 21 mins, 2 secs. Set 14 - 15 April 2004. UK.

2. World Speed Fitness Record (11 challenges):
1,750-metre swimming; 20-km running; 20-mile cycle; 2000 star jumps; 2000 sit-up crunches; weightlifting lifted 141 x 150 kgs; 1,400 hip flexors '5kg attached'; 2,326 metres carrying 40lb back pack; 10,000-metres rowing; 3km stepper, 500 alternate squat thrusts.
Time: 13 hrs, 59 mins, 55 secs. Set 6 - 7 Nov 2004. Germany.

3. World Fitness Champions Title Record (10 challenges):
2-mile + 21-metre swim; 20-mile row; 20¼-mile cross trainer; 10-mile speed march carrying 30lb back pack;
100¼-mile cycle; 550 star jumps; 3010 sit-up crunches, 300,000lb weightlifting 'upper body', 10¼ mile run; 505 hanging leg lifts.
Time: 17 hrs, 12 mins, 33 secs. Broken 27 Feb 2006. UK.

4. World Ultra Strength Speed Record (5 challenges):
833 step-ups carrying 40lb back pack '15 inch bench'; Rowed indoor 82.84 miles; cycled indoor 133.56 km; 130 back-of-hands push-ups carrying 40lb back pack; 220 shuttle sprints '30 ft' carrying 40lb back pack.
Time: 9 hrs, 55 mins, 02 secs. Set 13 May 2008. UK.

5. Most sit ups in 30 minutes with 50lb steel plate on chest total - 932.
Broken 2 July 2007. UK.

6. Multi Speed Fitness Record in 12 minutes: 123 press-ups; 108 sit-ups;114 one-arm push-ups; 90 squat thrusts; 33 para jumps; 102 back-of-hands push-ups.
Set 25 Sept 2002. UK.

7. Most full contact straight arm punches in 7 hrs 45 mins:
Total: 124,963 punches.
Broken 21 Jan 2008. UK.

8. 30-mile Arden cross country hill challenge walk carrying 40lb back pack:
Time: 7 hrs 45 mins. Set 13 Nov 2008. UK.

9. Special Forces Speed March (60-km/40-mile) carrying 55lb back pack over Brecon Beacons, Wales.
Time: 14 hrs 50 mins. Set 26 April 2003. Wales, UK.

10. Most back-of-hands push-ups in 30 mins:
Total: 1,386. Broken 8 Nov 2007. UK.

WORLD FITNESS ENDURANCE PROFILE / STATISTICS 2009

The following statistics lists some of most gruelling World Records I have beaten since 1987. These athletes certainly pushed me to my limits. Which I hold a lot of respect for them all. As mentioned on many occasions if it were not for these fitness endurance and martial arts boxing records, I would have directed my energy, possibly by breaking the law and ending up in jail. As I reflect on each of these records listed I can remember the many hours I spent training in the gym.

Some of the training sessions would last up to four hours of constant full contact sparring, bag work, circuit training, hill back pack speed marching and supportive shouting from my coaches and training team. I sometimes received worse injurys from the training sessions than actually attempting the challenges and titles , this was a great worry and a gamble, but I had to push myself to my limits, I needed to know mentally that I could break that fitness endurance records. I always say to my students "you have to go to the mountain, the mountain will not come to you". Point being you have to work hard, seek and go for the challenge.

{Please note some of these records have been beaten}

WORLD RECORD STRENGTH SPEED STAMINA PROFILE

The following statistics, details Athlete's World Records which have beaten by Paddy Doyle, since he started his career as a Endurance Athlete. These Athlete's have certainly pushed him to his limits. He has always stated that if it were not for sporting challenges which helped him to direct his energy and aggression, he would of certainly ended up in prison.

Some of the training sessions to prepare for these tough World Records, would last upto five hours of constant pure hard demanding physical training. The workouts with his training team and assistant coaches would involve full contact karate / boxing sparring, circuit training, hill back pack speed marching carrying 60 to 70 lb in weight. Mountain speed marching in North Wales and Scotland, and light weightlifting training combined with medicine ball strength training.

On some occasions whilst preparing for a challenge, he would sustain injurys which posed a threat when attempting a World Record. But that is the gamble he had to take to become the Worlds Number 1 World Endurance Champion, which is listed and recognised in the 2009 Guinness Book of World Records page 70.

Official World Record File of Athletes Beaten

Previous World Record And Title Holder	New World Record Result Beaten by Paddy Doyle {GB
Jeffrey Warwick {USA} 33,600 push ups in 24 hrs Set on 10 - 11th June 1998.	37,350 push ups in 24 hrs. Broken on 1st May 1989 UK
Adam Parsons {USA} 1,293,850 push ups in 1 year. Set from 1984 – 1985	1,500,230 push ups. Broken on Oct 1989 UK.
Garth Graham {GB} 1,866 squat thrusts in 1 hr. Set on 10th May 1988.	2,150 squat thrusts in 1 hr. Broken on 23 Feb 1990 UK
Colin Hewick {GB} 4,156 One arm push ups in 5 hrs Set on 8th July 1988.	5,260 One arm push ups in 5 hrs Broken on 6th May 1990 UK
Ashrita Furman {USA} 1,551 Para Jumps {burpees} 1 hr. Set on 13th March 1990.	1,619 Para Jumps {burpees} 1 hr Broken on 21 June 1991 UK
John Decker {GB} 5,550 One arm push ups in 5 hrs. Set on 13th May 1990.	7,643 One arm ups in 5 hrs Broken on 31st July 1990 UK
Patrick Doherty {GB} 1,777 Para Jumps {burpees} 1 hr Set on 25th Oct 1991.	1,840 Para jumps {burpees}1 hr Broken on 6th Feb 1994 UK

Ashrita Furman {USA}
64 mile walk, carrying
9 lb concrete brick in a
nominated hand.
Set on 13 - 14th June 1993

65 mile walk carrying 9 lb
concrete brick in nominated
hand. Broken on 3 – 4 Sept
1994. {Ireland}

Alan Rumbell {GB}
8,151 One arm push ups in 5 hrs.
Set on 26th June 1993.

8,794 One arm push ups in 5 hrs.
Broken on 12th Feb 1996 UK.

Jamie Borges {USA}
73 mile . 45 yards walk, carrying
9 lb concrete brick in a
nominated hand.
Set on 13 – 14 May 1996.

77 mile walk carrying 10 lb
concrete brick in a nominated
hand. Broken on 11 – 12
Feb 1998 UK.

Paul Wai Chung {Hong Kong}
3,552 squat thrusts in 1 hr.
Set on 21 Aug 1992.

3,743 squat thrusts in 1 hr.
Broken on 4th May 1998 UK.

Alistair Gillespie {GB}
1,051 back of hands push ups in 1 hr.
Set on 16 Feb 2001.

1,303 back of hands push ups
in 1 hr. Broken on 21 March
2001 UK.

Alves Filho {Brazil}
Most non stop Kumite Martial Arts
100 rounds in 3 hrs: 8 mins:
Won 26 fights by ippon
Won 50 by decision
Drew 24. Set on 22 March 1995.

Most non stop Kumite full contact
rounds in 3 hrs: 6 mins: Total 100.
Won 59 fights by ippon
Won 29 by decision. Drew 12.
Broken on 9 June 2002 UK.

Rob Powell {USA}
World Fittest Physical Fitness
Challenge Record. 11 cross training
challenges in 19 hrs: 17 mins:
Set in 2002.

11 cross training challenges in
18 hrs: 56 mins: 09 sec's:
Broken on 16 Feb 2005 UK

Ron Sarchian {USA}
15,089 punch strikes in 1 hr.
Set July 2005.

18,372 full contact punch
strikes in 1 hr. Broken on
19 Jan 2007 UK.

Rob Powell {USA}
World Fitness Champions
Title Record 10 cross training
challenges in 18 hrs: 15 mins: 02 sec's:

10 cross training challenge
Time 17 hrs: 12 mins: 33 sec
Broken on 27 Feb 2006 UK

Jim Hoover {USA}
333 boxing upper cuts in 1 min.
Set July 2002.

586 boxing upper cuts in 1
minute. Broken on 19
January 2007 UK.

James Clarke {USA}
Sit ups with 50 lb weight on
    chest. 5 min's
Sit ups with 50 lb weight on
    chest. 10 min's
Sit ups with 50 lb weight on
    chest. 15 min's
Sit ups with 50 lb weight on
    chest . 30 min's.
Records set 2006

Results. Carrying 50 lb steel
    plate on chest.
211 sit ups in 5 min's
351 sit ups in 10 min's

501 sit ups in 15 min's

932 sit ups in 30 min's

Records broken 2 July 2006 UK

Justin Carey {USA}
65 left arm throat strikes in 30 sec's
Set on 18 May 2006

67 throat strikes in 30 sec's.
Left arm only. Broken on
18th April 2007. World
Record Challenge Cup USA

Bruce Carey {USA
50 elbow strikes. Right arm only.
In 30 sec's. Set on 18th May 2006.

57 elbow strikes in 30 sec's. Left arm only. Broken on 18th April 2007. World Record Challenge Cup USA.

Bruce Carey {USA}
49 Right arm palm strikes in 30 sec's.

Set on 18 May 2006

60 palm strikes in 30 sec's. Right arm only. Broken on 18 April 2007. World Record Challenge Cup USA.

Bruce Carey {USA}
47 Left arm palm strikes in 30 sec's.
Set on 18 May 2006.

56 palm strikes in 30 sec's. Broken on 18 April 2007. World Record Challenge Cup USA.

Bruce Carey {USA}
51 right arm palm strikes in 30 sec's.
Set on 18 May 2006.

68 palm strikes in 30 sec's. Broken on 18 April 2007. World Record Challenge Cup USA.

Bruce Carey {USA}
54 left arm elbow strikes in 30 sec's.
Set on 18 May 2006.

66 left arm elbow strikes in 30 sec's. Broken on 18 April 2007. World Record Challenge Cup USA.

Bruce Carey {USA
Right arm throat strikes in 30 sec's.
Set on 18 May 2006.

68 right arm throat 61 strikes in 30 sec's. Broken on 18 April 2007. World Record Challenge Cup 2007.

Hart Carey {USA}
42 left arm elbow strikes in 30 sec's.
Set on 18 May 2006

54 left arm elbow strikes in 0 sec's Broken on 18 April 2007. World Record Challenge Cup 2007.

{Please note all martial arts strike records were broken at the Challenge Cup within 30 mins}

Doug Pruden {Canada}
1,781 back of hands push ups in 1 hr.
Set on 8 July 2005.

1,940 back of hands push ups in 1 hr. Broken on 8 Nov 2007 UK.

Attila Horvarth {Hungary}
4,656 squats in 1 hr.
Set on 30 Jan 2002.

4,708 squats in 1 hr. Broken on 8 Nov 2007 UK.

Ron Sarchian {USA}
5,545 full contact kicks in 1 hr.
Set 2007.

5,750 full contact martial arts kicks in 1 hr. Broken on 8 Nov 2007 UK.

Angelo Breaux {USA}
22,386 punch strikes in 1 hr.
Set 2007.

29,850 full contact punch strikes in 1 hr. Broken on 21 Jan 2008 UK.

Howard Smith {Wales}
121,471 punch strikes in 12 hrs.
Set 1988.

124,963 punch strikes in 7 hrs: 45 min's: Broken 21 Jan 2008 UK.

Rob Simpson {GB}
1,511 step ups carrying
40 lb back pack. In 1 hr.
Set Nov 2007.

1,619 step ups carrying 40 lb back pack, on 15 inch bench. Broken 13 May 2008 UK.

Suresh Joachim Arulanantham {Sri Lanka} 78. 7121 miles carrying 10 concrete brick in a nominated hand. Set on 11 – 12 Dec 1999. 80.372 miles carrying 10 lb concrete brick in a nominated hand. Broken on 21 May 2008 UK.

Source
Guinness Book of World Records
Registry of Record Holders www.recordholdersrepublic.co.uk
International Record Breakers Club www.recordholders.org

{Please note some of the records have since been beaten}

Summary

I believe a genuine champion is an athlete who can lose and come back stronger to regain his titles. To finally conclude, my personal ambitions have never been about making money. You are not remembered in life for how much money you made… you are remembered for what you have achieved in life.

BELIEVING IN YOURSELF

After competing in sport from the age of eight, my body is starting to feel the aches and pains. But when you love sporting challenges as much as I do, you accept it. It is part of the price you have to pay to be the World's Number One in your chosen sport. I know I would not be where I am today without my loyal training team and supporters.

When I instruct my self-defence and fitness endurance classes, I always express that the mind is far stronger than you could ever imagine. Anyone can achieve their chosen ambitions. For me it has never been about financial success, but just wanting to beat the best in the world in Endurance Athletics. And if any athlete takes one of my records off me, I will try my hardest to regain it. A genuine champion is an athlete who can accept a loss and come back stronger.

How long I can go on for remains to be seen, as I know I have beaten some of the world's toughest strength speed stamina records out there. I have never ducked a record which came under the fitness endurance category, which obviously had to be within my capabilities. On many occasions I have only been given five to seven days notice... and even 24-48 hours to attempt a World Record. Some of those records have included the Versa climber challenge, back-of-hands push-ups in one minute carrying a 40lb back pack, and the 10km speed march carrying a 40lb back pack.

Many athletes would want two to three months to prepare, but I gambled and it paid off. Some of those records have since been beaten easily, but those athletes possibly trained for up to three months. Analysing that in more detail, I suppose it shows the different levels of mental strength and physical fitness, plus having the confidence to step up to the wire and going for it.

Some athletes who have beaten my world records have been shouting their mouths off, saying that they will take all of my records off me, but they never seem to achieve it. They might take one or two records off me, but that is as far they get. To beat me totally, the athlete would have to beat all of my records before he could say he has beaten me. There is also one major factor… the fitness endurance records I am beating today are all held by athletes in their early thirties. I am forty-four years old. Since competing as an endurance athlete I have come across many bullshitters and space cadets whom I have approached and asked for a head-to-head challenge. And all I get is excuses.

To be the best at what you do, regardless of your career, you have to be hungry for success, have venom and the will to win. As I have stated already, my belief is that you are not remembered in life for how much money you earn. You are remembered in life for what you have achieved. Over the years I have had to self-finance my career. Having no money in your pocket hurts. I remember in the early days of attempting World Records that all I had was a fiver to my name.

When my mother was alive she used to help me as much as she could by supplying me with food.

I know what it's like to have no money, but I have learnt to get back on my feet and work hard to put food on my plate. I know if I keep trying at whatever I do, I will be able to earn a good wage one day. I'm not bothered about having lots of money, just being financially secure will be good enough.

Mark Dawes, the Director & National Coach, NFPS 2009, said:

'I have known Paddy for many years now and to me, Paddy is a remarkable man on many levels. It is obvious from his sporting and endurance achievements that he is an exceptional man, but if you ask him, he will say that he is simply a normal man who does exceptional things. And for me that is the part of him I have come to know, admire and respect. Outside of his public image Paddy is a very grateful and humble person who is quick to help others. He never takes anything for granted and never likes to feel like he is imposing on any one self, yet he will be one of the first to offer help and step up to the mark if asked to do so.

'In my professional capacity, I have had the privilege of meeting and working with some of the world's greatest achievers and some of the world's wealthiest people. One thing they all have in common is philanthropy and charity, the will to want to help others by their own efforts. It is this genuine and sincere altrusim for others that makes them successful. By giving, they know they will receive. For me, Paddy is one of the greatest and yet unrecognized givers in the UK today. He gives everything so that he can be an inspiration for others to follow. Paddy's focus and determination is built upon the very foundations that make all successful individuals. To me he is a great man. He is rich in kindness and wealthy in spirit. He is a beacon of light that many can draw strength and encouragement from. He is the lighthouse in the sea of despair, but most of all he is my friend and that is a gift you can't buy.'

GREAT TIMES AND WHAT'S NEXT

Since embarking on a long tough journey of breaking fitness endurance records, I have had the pleasure of meeting some great individuals, such as Norris McWhirter, founder of the Guinness book of Records; Roy Castle, World Record Holder and BBC Record Breakers presenter; Chris Akabussi, former Olympic athlete, Ashrita Furman, multiple Guinness World Record Holder, and the Great Throwdini, who holds many world knife-throwing records... a man I totally respect.

My loyal team of trainers, partners and medical advisers have backed me all the way and been invaluable to me. I would like to go for a few more World Records this year and then consider my options. If there is one thing I have learnt throughout my career as an athlete, it is that the older you get the more time the body takes to heal. So before I start training again I am going to make sure that I am one hundred percent fit. I am presently recovering from a lower back injury which has halted my plans to attempt endurance records I have my eyes on. I am having regular treatment and hope it soon repairs itself. My next challenge is to complete my

Winter Mountain Leader Award, which is very hard to pass. Fingers crossed, my back should be better by the time I decide to go for my Winter Mountain Leader assessment.

So what does the future hold for me? The first thing is to stay out of trouble and only help those who need it, then to pass my personal fitness trainer's course, climbing instructors course , and teach up-and-coming athletes how to break world records. It would be a great pity if I never passed on my knowledge and skills to those who want to learn. Rest assured… there's still plenty of gas left in the tank.

About the Author

Since the age of 8 yrs of age, he was introduced to Judo competing at junior level, winning bronze and silver medals at numerous Midlands judo championships. Coming .from a broken home made him more determined and hungry to succeed. Any sport which he took up he always gave 100% winning more medals.

His aggression was channelled through sport however he was still getting into trouble with law. The Parachute Regiment and the thought of breaking Fitness and Endurance Records, made Paddy more focused, wanting to be the Worlds number I.

Since May 1987 he has clocked up a career total of 172. Course, Regional, National, British, European World strength speed stamina records; 1,940 back of bands push ups in 1 hour, 29,850 full contact punches in 1 hour, 932 sit ups carrying 50 lbs weight on chest in 30 minutes, 1,500,230 push ups in a calender year averaging 4000 per day.

Pure Grit exposes the true Paddy Doyle, his fallouts with his fellow competitors, his toughest and most demanding World Fitness Endurance Records, and what makes him tick mentally.

Printed in the United Kingdom by
Lightning Source UK Ltd., Milton Keynes
141183UK00002B/2/P